Losing Weight after Pregnancy

Losing Weight *after* Pregnancy

A Step-by-Step Guide to Fitness and Health

Elisabeth Bing and Libby Colman

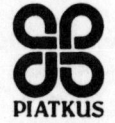

PIATKUS

© 1995 Elisabeth Bing and Libby Colman

This edition first published in Great Britain in 1995 by
Judy Piatkus (Publishers) Limited
5 Windmill Street, London W1P 1HF

The moral right of the authors has been asserted

*A catalogue record for this book
is available from the British Library*
ISBN 0 7499 1433 5

Designed by Paul Saunders
Illustrations by Judith Deming

Typeset by Computerset, Harmondsworth
Printed and bound in Great Britain by
Bookcraft Ltd, Midsomer Norton, Avon

CONTENTS

	Acknowledgements	vi
	Introduction: 'Is This Really Me?'	1
1	Childbearing and Self-Image	9
2	The First Five Days	29
3	The Next Five Weeks	53
4	Losing Weight While Breast-Feeding	81
5	Weight Change Over the Childbearing Year	101
6	Putting It All Together	123
	Helpful Organisations	136

ACKNOWLEDGEMENTS

We could not have written this book without the help of the many women we interviewed, questioned, either personally or by phone, and the women who allowed us to tape our conversations with them and who were infinitely patient, helpful, and full of enthusiasms and ideas that we could incorporate into this book. We would like to thank them all for the hours they gave us.

And we also want to thank our editor, Jenny Cox, not only for initially suggesting the idea of this book, but above all for supporting us with ideas, advice, changes, and immeasurable patience during the writing of this book.

ELISABETH BING
LIBBY COLMAN

INTRODUCTION

Is This Really Me?

When you look at yourself in the mirror in the early weeks after having a baby, you may find yourself saying. 'Is this really me?' Even if your weight is only a few pounds over normal, your face and figure will be different from the way they were before. Like women all over the world and down through the ages, you gained weight during pregnancy and will lose much of it in the first two months after your baby is born. In the meantime, you wonder if you will ever get back to feeling like yourself again.

You would have gained and lost weight during this year even if you had not changed the amount of food you ate. In pregnancy and after the birth, your body goes through many startling transformations, some of which you can see and most of which are invisible. You knew that your belly would grow large and that you would be eating for two. Did you also know that you would put your calories to new uses and that you would store fat, water, and protein in different ways during pregnancy than at other times of your life? Your body and many of its organs and even individual cells grew to unprecedented size and have to shrink again now that the baby is born. While you were pregnant, you lost your waistline and discovered your uterus. Your body built and sustained another human being; you had the unsettling experience of being kicked from within. Now you can watch your baby grow fat from sucking at your breast, for you've gained the capacity to create milk. All these changes in our body are hard to believe!

Even though the amazing events of gestation and lactation affect the details of your cellular life as well as the way you use the food you eat, the basic truths about weight control remain the same: if you want to lose weight, you must either exercise more or eat less—and you should do both. We will tell you about the special concerns regarding diet and exercise for the postnatal woman so that you can establish healthy patterns for yourself and your new baby.

While we will deal primarily with practical matters, it is important to remember that behind all the issues of diet and exercise lie the deeper issues of human relationships. In order to be able to do a good job taking care of others you have to feel that you are being taken care of yourself. When you feel emotionally supported by your family and friends, you are more able to relax while you feed your baby and remember to be careful when feeding yourself.

You did not become a mother in a vacuum. You belong to a society and to a family. Just as you needed your family when you were a child, it is important that you seek out other people with whom you can share the special concerns of this time of life. Your parents, your partner, and your friends who have already had babies will be especially important to you now. We encourage you to spend time with others who share your values and dreams about parenting.

Is This Really Me?

Your weight is influenced not only by the dictates of your physiology, but also by the meaning of food in your life. Psychologist/author Kim Chernin suggests that eating disorders (both overeating and undereating) are related to the mother–daughter relationship, particularly to unconscious feelings that come up for a daughter who is in the process of surpassing her mother's success in life. If Chernin's theory is correct, we should expect that women should have trouble with food when they become mothers. It could be that women who gain weight after they have a baby instead of following the more natural pattern of losing it gradually while breast-feeding are influenced by ambivalence about the mother–daughter relationship. You are still the daughter of your own mother even though you are now the mother of your new child. Confusion and competition are inherent in the situation.

Food takes on new and complex meanings in pregnancy and the postnatal period because you are creating and nurturing another person as well as yourself. Many of us equate food and love. You may not feel as though this is true for you, but think about it for a moment. Eating is at the heart of taking care of others and feeling taken care of yourself. In the early weeks, the parent–child bond centres around the breast or bottle, for the newborn is awake and alert for short periods and must eat during much of that time in order to consume the calories it needs for all the growing it must do. When you are a new mother, it is especially important that you do not become emotionally deprived or starved, because your main job as a mother will be to nurture and sustain your baby. Your emotional well-being will be an important factor in your ability to eat and exercise sensibly after the birth.

Most people want to be able to love deeply and well and to put the needs of others before their own. This is especially true for you because you have just become a mother. You may want to sing to your baby and rock him to sleep and take time to kiss his tummy and tickle his toes, but in reality sometimes you are too exhausted or depleted to live up to your hopes for yourself.

How do you find the time or energy to pay attention to your own body and its needs? That is a central question of parenting, one that has both symbolic and practical aspects.

When you have just had a baby, you are busy adjusting to change. You have to get up in the middle of the night to feed your baby; your personal time is often interrupted by his or her cries; you may have to tend to the baby's needs when you would rather be socialising with other adults or doing something for yourself. Your eating and sleeping patterns and many other of your life rhythms have been disrupted, and yet you must make sure you get all the nutrients you and your baby need and you must pay particular attention to the vulnerable state of your own body.

The physical changes of childbearing are so dramatic that even years later, women talk about them as though they happened yesterday. Everyone we have talked with about losing weight after having a baby has had a story to tell. We have collected many of these stories from women who have shared with us their intimate experiences with their bodies

Is This Really Me?

and also their outlook on their lives. As we listened to others, our own postnatal experiences came back to us vividly. Each childbirth is unique, and yet each new mother is participating in a universal biological reality.

You are probably reading this book because you want to know if there are ways you can speed up the process of getting your figure back without jeopardising your health or your baby's well-being. Of course you want to be mature and unselfish, but you may have doubts about whether you can accept your new burdens gracefully and whether it is normal to feel weighed down by your new responsibilities. You want to be as slender as you were before pregnancy but may feel guilty about such a selfish desire when your child is the most important thing just now. You are not alone. You can identify with the women we've interviewed because they have been through it. Their stories will teach you that this is a temporary life stage. Even if it feels overwhelming to you now, the postnatal period will pass. Your life, your body, and your baby will grow more familiar to you in time.

Many women find their weight fluctuates a bit throughout their lives. Some women report predictable changes during their monthly cycle, when premenstrual water retention causes them to feel heavy and bloated. Childbearing is even more extreme. The water retention of pregnancy and the hormonal dip after giving birth are exaggerations of the ups and downs of a monthly cycle. The weight gain of pregnancy included changes in *your* body that were a necessary part of sustaining a child. Your figure needed the extra reserves it stored during pregnancy in anticipation of breast-feeding, a process that draws on the fat stored in various parts of your body.

You may never quite return to being as you were before, because you are in a different phase of your life. Even when you achieve the same weight you had before getting pregnant, you are deeply different on a psychological and social level, and often on a physical level as well. You have created and become responsible for the life of another human being. You are a mother. Your body will reflect your new state to a greater or lesser degree.

We want to caution you to be accepting of the body changes that are a natural part of the childbearing year. The most important thing just now is to keep up your energy so that you can fulfil the demands of your new role and enjoy this very special time in your life.

1
Childbearing and Self-Image

In the postnatal period, your body's physical changes may be more frustrating to you than they were during pregnancy. Why is your body still so different? Why can't you get into your favourite blue jeans? When will you ever feel like yourself again?

You may also feel a letdown from the way people are treating you. Pregnant women are special and get extra attention. What about new mums? Does anyone even know that you have a baby if you go out by yourself? You are different, but the reason for it is not as conspicuous as when you were pregnant.

The physical changes of pregnancy and the postnatal period have a profound effect on your sense of yourself. How you feel inside yourself may be more important than how you actually appear to others. To you it may seem that your body has changed a great deal, even though your friends assure you that you seem to be the same as before.

If you have ever considered yourself fat, or if others considered you pudgy as a child, you may find that the weight gain of pregnancy activates an underlying image of yourself as overweight, which can be disturbing. But think about the way your body changed during pregnancy. Your weight gain entailed more than a neat little round belly and larger breasts. You became rounder everywhere, because your body tissue retained water as part of the healthy process of gestation. Even the shape of your face changed. If you preferred to think of yourself as fashionably slender and elegant, you probably did not like what you saw.

Pregnancy always seems to go beyond our expectations and take us farther away from our usual experience than we anticipate. You may even have thought, Surely this is not me. If you felt that way, it is time to remember that the weight you put on in pregnancy was creative growth, not obesity. If you have been happy with your weight all your life, it will be easy to realise that the pregnant you was not a fat you. In fact, much if not all the weight you put on during pregnancy had very little to do with excess fat. It was made up of the foetus, the organs that support its growth, and energy stored for childbirth and lactation.

Let's break down the factors that contributed to the total amount of weight gained during pregnancy. The foetus and the organs that directly support it (the placenta, the amniotic fluid, and the enlarged uterus) added up to 16–20 pounds (7.25–9 kg). Then why did you have to gain an additional 5 or 10 pounds (2.3–4.5 kg)? Because you had to do more than just carry the baby and its support system. You also had to supply the basis for further growth and maintenance of both yourself and the baby. The food you ate every day during pregnancy was immediately used to create new cells in your body and in the baby's. In addition, some of it was stored in cells throughout your body for future use. The extra water, protein, and fat tend to accumulate especially in the tissue of your hips and thighs, your upper arms, and your breasts.

It may be hard to believe that the mother's figure is too important for the well-being of the foetus, but study after study has shown that the best assurance of the healthy development of the foetus is the mother's pattern of weight gain. In the 1960s, doctors tried to keep women's gain under 20 pounds (9 kg), and they enforced their goal by monitoring it carefully. A few doctors and many grandmothers-to-be still believe that it is 'bad' to gain more than 15 or 20 pounds (6.8 or 9 kg) during pregnancy. They couldn't be more wrong. Medical evidence shows that women who are at a healthy weight before pregnancy should gain 25–35 pounds (11.3–15.9 kg) to grow a well-nourished, full-sized baby. Women who are at a low or normal weight before pregnancy and don't gain 20 pounds (9 kg) are at a much greater risk of giving birth to a baby who is of a low birth weight, and low-birth-weight babies are at risk of many medical complications.

Christina, a woman in her late thirties who had always wanted to be pregnant, told us:

> 'I didn't understand before I experienced it myself. I didn't understand why people were so upset with their bodies during pregnancy. I thought they looked absolutely gorgeous. Then I got pregnant and for the first three months I felt so lousy I thought: Why not adopt? I was so miserable I just felt bad about everything that had anything to do with my body.'

Christina's reaction came as a surprise to her, but it was perfectly normal. She hadn't realised how complete the changes in her body would be.

If you had been told to put on 25 pounds (11.3 kg) any other year of your life, you might have had to work at it by taking food supplements, but during pregnancy it probably happened spontaneously. When you're pregnant, your body metabolises calories more efficiently than at other times. More than calories, you need nutrients and fluids for a healthy pregnancy, in order to convert them into amniotic fluid, extra blood, and fuel for the growth of your baby.

Water retention is the most variable factor contributing to weight gain during pregnancy. Some women retain a great deal of fluid and others relatively little, just as some women gain 5 pounds (2.3 kg) or more from premenstrual water retention and others gain only a pound or two. You may not like your puffy look, but, in general, increased body water is related to healthier babies. You will probably retain more water later in the pregnancy. It seems to be part of our biology, part of the process of creating a body that can sustain a baby's life, to store extra water along with fat and protein.

Our feminine propensity to plump up our body tissue during pregnancy is an essential part of our maternal body and is meant to help us survive and take care of our babies. Some of that extra padding is converted to energy for labour. Much more of it will be used for the demands of the postnatal period, especially for creating milk and to sustain breast-feeding.

It is normal to feel that your body is unfamiliar in the postnatal period; you are still in the midst of profound changes. But no matter how different it seems, it is your own. Your body is adjusting to unfamiliar demands. Be patient; it will take a while to adjust to your image of yourself and realise that 'mother' is really you, not that other woman, the one who raised you.

Here are the words of Gayle, a woman who was trying to understand the changes in her body:

'I was interested to see how my whole sense of my size was off kilter after my baby was born. I didn't have a concept of how big I was. I had worn size ten before getting pregnant. I went to buy jeans and tried on the eighteens because that is how big I thought I'd be. I was thrilled to discover that the eighteens were way too big. Even the fourteens were loose on me, but the twelves were a little tight until about six months after giving birth.'

The physical changes of childbearing are so profound that a perfectly normal and psychologically healthy woman might not have a realistic sense of her own body size. Children know that their bodies are growing all the time. They pay a lot of attention to their size and to their height relative to their friends. They love to measure themselves against the mark on the doorjamb that they made the year before. Grown-ups seem to expect their bodies to remain more static. Isn't that what is implied by the expression 'grown up'?

But of course our bodies continue to change throughout adulthood. When we exercise more, we develop larger muscle mass. When we eat less, we have smaller tummies. As we age, we sag. There is a lot we can do to control our body shape, but we are not plastic dolls that stay the same for decades. The childbearing year reminds us of just how fluid our bodies are, for change is more sudden and dramatic then than at other times in adulthood.

Melanie shared her experience with us:

'I joined a new mothers' group after I had my second baby. I found that many of the women were unhappy with their bodies. I said, "Give yourself time! How many kids are you going to have? Relax and enjoy pregnancy, nursing, and parenting. This is a temporary, time-limited stage of your life."

'One day the whole group went shopping together. They all bought new dresses that fit their present figures, and all felt so much better about themselves.'

As an experienced mother, Melanie was more patient than the others in her group. She knew that her baby, her body, and her life-style would become more organised over time. She also recognised that her friends felt a lot better about themselves when they were well groomed. It is worth looking good even in a temporary stage!

You will need some time to integrate the changes in your body with your usual sense of yourself. Inside that changed body is still the old you as well as the changing you; you are still an individual adult as well as an expectant or new mother. Pregnancy and the postnatal period are important stages in your life, but not everything. This is part of who you are, but not all of you. It may feel alien or it may be the experience you have been waiting for. A woman we'll call Marcy told us:

'I know some women feel like a beached whale when they are pregnant. I never felt that way. I was awkward, but I knew it was because of the baby and I just found the whole experience fascinating. I liked watching the changes.'

Painters and sculptors have always seen the beauty of pregnancy and breast-feeding. From the earliest times you will see the full figure of childbearing women represented in sculpture and art. Notice that you never see a skinny Madonna. Realising that you are part of this universal process can be exciting and reassuring.

You may wonder whether your partner still finds you attractive. He should understand that you are not really fat, even if you have put on an unusual amount of weight with the pregnancy. Many men are thrilled by the 'glow of pregnancy'. Listen to Alexis's words:

'Lots of men told me how great I looked all through my pregnancy, even at the end, when I had gained 3 stone 3 pounds (20.4 kg). My husband was particularly interested in my new shape.'

No one expects you to look the same just now, but they know what you may forget–that the most conspicuous changes in your body are temporary. It will be a great help for you if your friends and your partner can reassure you that they recognise you as the lovely woman they have known even in the midst of the extraordinary changes going on in your body as well as in your life. Margaret's partner helped her with this even though he preferred her figure before pregnancy. As she told us:

'My husband wants lots of children and is thrilled when I'm pregnant and seems to think I'm most beautiful then. He doesn't seem to notice my body changes after giving birth. He just wants me to be happy. I know he likes thin women, but he thinks I'm doing fine.'

Some men are genuinely delighted by the fuller figure, and some are turned off by it. We cannot predict how the people close to you will react, but we know that women with supportive partners feel better about themselves and their babies. We hope that the two of you will be sensitive to each other's feelings. Nadia was very lucky:

'I have a fabulous husband, which makes a difference. He didn't say, "Oh, finally you have a bosom," or anything like that. Once I asked him, "What if I got fat? Would you still like me?" and she said, "I'd just have more to explore!"'

Sometimes a man and a woman have difficulties in adjusting to the woman's changed body during lovemaking. This is a practical situation that can be solved with love and creative problem solving. If you feel that you are not desirable, you may need extra romance from your partner to help you feel attractive. This is a wonderful time in your life to have someone around you who keeps reminding you that you are a desirable woman. Again, Nadia talks about her marriage:

> 'After my son was born, my husband made me feel that being a mother hadn't taken over all the areas of my life. He made me feel that I was still an attractive, sexual woman and that I looked great!'

Your health, diet, and exercise during your pregnancy were the basis of your health and weight and body tone now, in the postnatal period. They were also the basis for the growth and nutritional status of your infant at birth. A solid foundation in pregnancy is the best possible condition for creating a healthy baby, staying healthy and vigorous yourself, and regaining a figure you recognise as your own within the first year of giving birth. How much you gained in pregnancy seems less important than how well you gained it.

Medical research suggests that British women generally get most of the nutrients they need from their normal diet. Nevertheless, you probably took a vitamin and mineral supplement during pregnancy. The foetus took its important nutrients from the fresh foods that you consumed daily as they passed from your digestive tract into your blood and through the placenta into the baby's blood, but your doctor did not want to risk any possibility that you or the baby might not get all the building blocks for your bodies. You needed extra calories, extra protein, iron, calcium, and nutrients then just as you do now. It is best to get them from a good diet, but it is essential that you get them, so be sure to take the supplement if your health-care giver recommends it.

If you put on a lot of weight, or if your abdomen stretched an unusual amount, the chances are that you will have a harder time getting your figure back. If you did not exercise during the pregnancy, and lost muscle tone, you may have added inches whether or not you came away with added pounds. You will probably have some loose skin that does not go away and you may find that your stretch marks are still visible to you, but they will fade until they are hardly noticeable to others, even in your favourite bikini. If you are a perfectionist, you may prefer to keep your body hidden, but even when you are in a bathing suit, others will be unlikely to notice the difference. Some women even consider their stretch marks a badge of courage, the proud remnant of their motherhood.

Sandy was 5'7" (171 cm) tall and weighed 8 stone 3 pounds (52.2 kg) before she became pregnant. She told us:

> 'It was important for me to put the baby before my own appearance. I have moved into a new stage of my life and I don't have to look like a boy anymore. Even at

the same weight, my body has changed. My hips are wider, as though from the bones opening up at childbirth. I have a womanly figure for the first time in my life.'

Sandy was in her mid-thirties and ready for these changes.

You may find that you have some trouble keeping a positive self-image through the final stage of pregnancy and in the period that follows. Our culture stresses an ideal female body that has a flat stomach, long legs, and small breasts. This is certainly not the body type of a pregnant or postnatal woman! We realise that it is often hard to reconcile fantasy and reality. We are all structured differently; so much about weight depends on your body type, which is influenced by your genetics and your metabolism as well as your temperament. There is only so much that you can reasonably do to control your shape to fit a social image of beauty.

Look at the silhouettes of women's figures on page 22. Which one looks most like a good mother? Probably the plump one. Is it also the one that you would choose as the ideal image of yourself? Is your image of a 'mum' consistent with your image your true self? You should also think about whether your ideal image for yourself is realistic as long as you are lactating. Does it fit your current body type and lifestyle?

Were you very thin or very heavy before you became

Losing Weight After Pregnancy

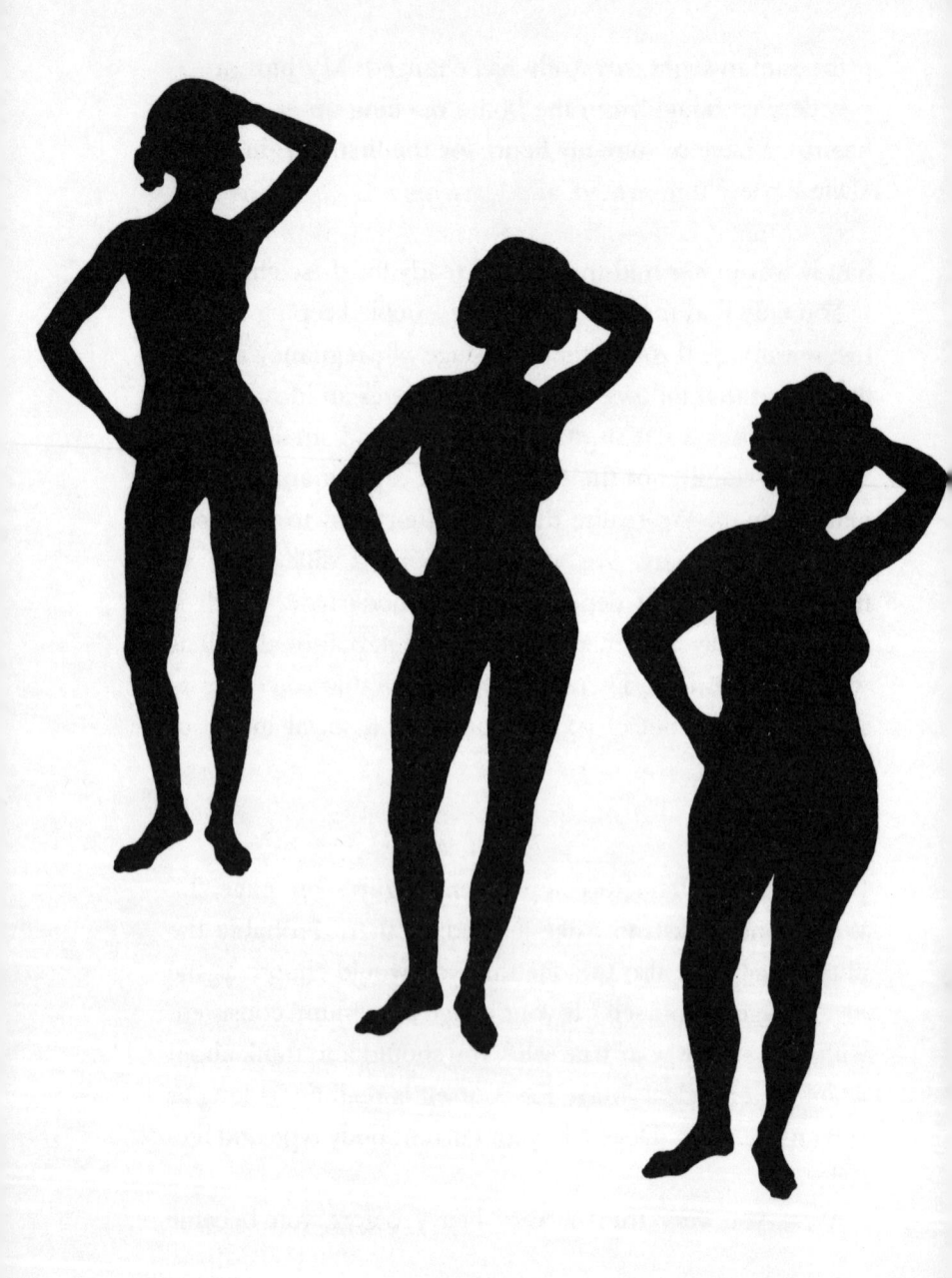

Childbearing and Self-Image

pregnant? In order to stay energetic during the childbearing year and to create a healthy child, an underweight woman has to gain more than an overweight woman. If you have always been thin-armed and flat-chested, your pregnant and postnatal body will be more alien to you than if you have always been 'pleasingly plump'.

If you feel your figure is more maternal now, that might either feel wonderful or troubling to you. In mythology, the Amazons, women warriors, were said to have cut off their right breasts because they got in the way in archery. Similarly, the comfortable figure of a breast-feeding mum may be an impediment in the competitive workplace that thinks in terms of 'lean and mean'. You may feel as though the silhouette on the right is fine for someone else, but does it feel like you?

As you reflect upon your feelings about how a mother should look, you must also consider your actual body type. Do you tend toward retaining water and putting on weight during certain parts of your menstrual cycle? Or are you trim and athletic? What kind of metabolism do you have? You must reconcile your actual physical type with your ideal figure and take into consideration the temporary influences of childbearing.

We hear people say that they are afraid they will 'let themselves go', as though they assume that mothers don't take as good care of themselves as other people do. Sally was worried about that:

'I watched a friend start to regain her sense of herself

as a woman after she had a baby, but then she just sort of let go of her old self and let "mother" take over her image of herself. She had two more babies right in a row and never got her figure back in between.'

In studies of postnatal weight gain that have been done around the world, scientists have determined that women retain an average of two pounds (0.9 kg) of weight after each baby. Don't let that statistic alarm you. It is based primarily on women from developing countries who were undernourished to begin with. The weight gain is an important positive part of their reproductive lives. Well-nourished middle-class women in this country cannot realistically learn what to expect for themselves from this data. You are an individual who can shape much of your own life and your experience will be unique.

In the 'old days' when motherhood almost always marked the end of a career outside the home, women were sometimes cut off from other arenas of personal development and retreated into a martyred role. Feeling isolated and unhappy, such women became depressed. Perhaps this is the origin of the cultural myth that mothers are dowdy. If you associate motherhood with the end of personal opportunities for growth in other areas, you might indeed 'let yourself go'.

Depression is still more common among postnatal women than in the general population, and weight gain is often associated with depression. Some women with special emotional issues about motherhood get into a negative cycle of weight gain and low self-esteem but this is not the

Childbearing and Self-Image

experience of most contemporary middle-class mothers. If you find yourself withdrawing from the world, watching an unusual (for you) amount of TV, or eating in unhealthy patterns, it may be symptomatic of depression. Don't fade away. Reach out for support. There are ways to address your needs, even while you are taking care of a baby.

There is no reason at all why you should become unattractive after you have had a baby. Women with children can be as conscious of their appearance as any others. Think of Princess Di or Meryl Streep or any of dozens of Hollywood stars who are absolutely gorgeous mothers. Marathon runners and other athletes who continue to compete after they bear children do not differ noticeably from others in their class.

Of course movie stars and world-class athletes are exceptional. They must be more careful than the rest of us not to carry extra weight. They doubtless find, as many working mothers do, that they do not have as much time to relax into the soft, comfortable, cuddly parts of motherhood as they would like. This can be a terrible conflict for them or for you, and it is often reflected in concerns about weight.

Your motivation to be slender does not necessarily change just because you are becoming a mother, but you may find that after the baby is born, you do not have the time or energy to do what you should to lose the extra weight you gained while you were carrying the baby. Your schedule may be too full and chaotic for you to exercise regularly or to pay a great deal of attention to diet. You must keep up your energy and make sure that you get all the nutrition you need for the demands of your new life. Movie stars usually have help shopping and cooking and baby-sitting to free them to eat properly and find time to get to exercise class. You may not be so fortunate. It may take you several months to work out a routine that allows you to take care of the baby, manage your home smoothly, and pay attention to your own eating and exercise. Be patient with the changes that are characteristic of your present stage. You will become more organised with time.

The extra weight that is stored to serve as backup for breast-feeding, the broader hips and enlarged breasts that create such a comfortable lap for the infant, are just the things that make it impossible for you to fit back into your work clothes or keep you from being able to button your favourite jeans. These conspicuous changes of childbearing are a necessary part of gestation and breast-feeding, but need not dominate your life forever.

Many women these days are well into their thirties when they decide to have a child, and they may worry whether they will have a harder time regaining their pre-pregnant figures. A woman of thirty-nine who exercised long before she became pregnant may have excellent muscle tone and regain her shape fairly quickly after having a baby.

There is no medical evidence that weight gain during pregnancy or lactation is influenced by age. Pre-pregnancy weight, body type, eating patterns, and amount of activity are far more important factors. However, in your late thirties you will have to work harder to regain your preferred weight after having a baby, because with age it takes more dedication or will power to remain slender.

Weight gain is a normal part of aging. We are not referring to the difference between a woman of twenty-five and one of thirty, but obviously the bodies of a woman at eighteen and one at forty-two are quite different. In fact, the same woman having her first baby in her early twenties and her second at forty may find her body responds differently to the two experiences—not only because of her age, but also because once muscles and tissue have been stretched during one pregnancy, they will stretch again more quickly the next time, whether you are twenty-six or thirty-six. This does not necessarily mean that you will be significantly fatter when you have recovered from childbearing.

Lorraine compared her experience at ages twenty-three and thirty-eight:

> 'I had my second child fifteen years after my first. I still had that sense of pregnancy as a miracle, but I also had some shortness of breath and more swelling of the ankles that I didn't have when I was younger. But both times I remember being tired and sleeping more than usual. Both times I kept physically active right up to the end and got my regular weight back within the first year.'

Throughout the childbearing year, it is important that you listen to the messages of your body. Your experience will not be exactly like anyone else's. It depends on your unique metabolism, on your diet, the rate of growth of your child, and your level of activity. Extraordinary new demands are being made on your internal supply of energy during pregnancy and lactation. No matter what your age or body type, you will have to experiment to find a life-style that works for you.

If your ideal is thinner than your body type allows, childbearing may help you relax into acceptance of your figure, for now you are a mum.

Ruth expressed a common experience:

'After I had my baby, I was afraid I would never get my life or my eating patterns back to normal, not just my body. Sleep deprivation does a lot of funny things to your psyche. I thought maybe I'd be like that the rest of my life, but I found out that it was time-limited. It passed.'

Some of you may discover that childbearing is a good time to bring your weight down, perhaps not right after the baby is born, but in the year or so after. You will be paying more attention to nutrition because of the needs of the foetus and then of the baby if you are breast-feeding, and this attention to your diet may help you establish very healthy habits that ultimately lead to a trim figure.

2
The First Five Days

These first five days after the birth are extraordinary, especially in the ways your body loses weight. One of Elisabeth's students called her a day after she had given birth and said, 'I look like I'm still pregnant. What's wrong with me?' Elisabeth assured her that the only thing wrong was the unfortunate circumstance that she had forgotten this basic truth: that her body would not magically snap back into shape.

You may have assumed that your body would feel familiar to you immediately after the birth. A few women return to normal quickly, but for most it takes more than days or weeks of adjusting. Muscle tissue and skin are extremely elastic and will regain tone, but the process may take longer than you expected. If you think of how far your skin and muscle had to stretch to accommodate your baby, you will realise that there is no way that they could spring right back to their former shape.

Traditionally, women have spent weeks recuperating from childbirth. Many Asian cultures talk of postnatal woman 'doing the month.' All the people around her acknowledge her vulnerability. For a month, the new mother receives special treatment. She is not expected to participate in the work of the community and she may even be privileged to receive chicken to eat!

In our country before World War II, new mothers often stayed in nursing homes for ten days. Nowadays you are probably at home within three days (or five days if you had a caesarean section) and you may not have help for your physical needs, for the house or for the baby. Never forget that your health is of a very high priority. These first five days, you should not be alone for long and you must be pampered if at all possible.

It is far better to be among loving and understanding caregivers than to be among strangers. Unfortunately, your family may think that you are fine and fully recovered when you are actually still quite shaky. They may expect you to run the house and to handle your life as before—plus, of course, take care of the baby.

If you don't have anyone who can stay home from work to be with you, see if you can find a special agency that trains caregivers especially to help new mothers in the early days after childbirth. They may understand what inexperienced family members do not, that you are unusually fatigued and needful, but not sick.

If you are alone in the early period after your baby is born, try to get plenty of rest and eat well. You especially cannot afford the fatigue and irritability that come with poor nutrition!

You will find that if your loved ones show sincere concern for you in the early days after you have a baby, if you know that you are well cared for, you will have an easier time

The First Five Days

learning to take care of your baby and you will be more conscientious establishing healthy eating patterns for yourself. But don't let anyone nag you about your eating! Nagging brings out the worst in us all.

There is time enough in your life to get to your ideal weight. Do not do it at the expense of your own or your child's health. Think about the demands of your new life and be realistic about what you can do. Most new mothers find their life extremely demanding. It is important that you have energy to sustain the demands being made on your body during this period so that you can experience it as a joyous transition rather than an overwhelming stress.

You have been through a major physical event. It is not an illness and, unless you had a caesarean section, it was not an operation, but even healthy and vigorous women need to rest after the wear and tear of childbirth, just as athletes have to rest after a major sporting event. Think about how professional football players spend their time after a game. They soak in a hot bath and go to the physiotherapist. A woman can also expect to need a period of recovery from the vigorous experience she has just been through.

Now is the time to get your loved ones to help you toward your goal of eating well and regaining your figure at the same time. Take advantage of your period of recovery after childbirth to let your family help you with the grocery shopping, meal planning, and meal preparation. In your first days at home from the hospital, let others bring you nutritious snacks and make sure you have healthy food in the house.

Many women forget to step on a scale during the first five days after giving birth because they are more involved in other things—the sensations in their bodies, the fascinating baby, excited friends and family. Some sensible women refuse to step on a scale until their six-week checkup. But you may be curious.

If you do check your weight right away, beware. Many of the pounds gained in the pregnancy are still stored in your body's cells and will be lost gradually and naturally over weeks or even months. The changes of pregnancy entail far more than simply a baby in your uterus, and your body needs to do more than give birth to the baby to lose that extra weight.

The average woman loses 12–17 (5.4–7.7 kg) pounds at childbirth. This total is made up of:

the baby	6–8 pounds (2.72–3.6 kg)
the placenta	1–2 pounds (0.4536–0.9 kg)
amniotic fluid	2–3 pounds (0.9–1.4 kg)
blood and other body fluids lost at birth	3–4 pounds (1.4–1.8 kg)

The exact amounts are highly variable. Our point is that you lose only about half of a normal weight span of pregnancy in your first hours after giving birth.

We've even heard some reports from women who claim that they weighed as much the morning after they gave birth as they had the morning before—women like Gloria, who told us:

'When I stepped on the scale three hours after my nine-pound baby was born, I weighed only two and a half pounds less than I had the night before. How was that possible?'

We're not sure how that was possible. We think experiences like Gloria's are based on quirks of scales or meals or other momentary oddities. Perhaps she received and retained a significant amount of intravenous fluids during labour. But the norms are clear. You probably won't lose as much as you expected, but you will lose quite a bit.

In addition to the evidence on the scale, you must also confront the evidence of your abdomen and of your waistline. There is no baby in there, but you don't have a flat tummy, either. Your uterus is still enlarged. It will be shrinking down into your pelvic cavity over the next two weeks, but at first it still rises above the pubic bone, almost up to your navel. It needs time to shrink back into its old place. Your doctor or nurse-midwife will feel its size and check its gradual return to normal every time you have a checkup.

Your skin is likely to be loose and still quite stretched out. Even your muscles may feel as though they have been through an ordeal. Here are Melissa's words:

'Right after the baby was born, I felt tired and achy all over, especially in my shoulders, neck, and back, like I'd had a big workout. More than anything, I just wanted a bath. That first day, I felt like I was still pregnant, but when I put my hand down on my abdomen, it felt flatter. I was eager to get out of bed but then I felt shaky when I tried to walk.'

It's a lot to adjust to! Don't despair; it took you nine months to get this way and may take that many to return to 'yourself'.

You will urinate a lot from the second to the fifth day, getting rid of two or three quarts of water that you retained in cells throughout your body. Some women have even more than that. Maggie's experience is not too uncommon:

'My weight goes up five pounds (2.2 kg) when I ovulate just from water retention, so you can imagine what pregnancy was like for me. I had so much fluid I could poke and squish it on the tops of my feet. My shoe size went from size 5 to size $6^1/_2$.'

That much fluid will not be expelled in a single day!

In this very early period, you will have a discharge, called lochia, from your vagina. It seems like a menstrual period but is part of the process of your uterus healing at the place where the placenta had been attached. In the four weeks or more it takes for this process, you will lose the equivalent of half a pound (0.23 kg) in weight just from passing lochia.

If after five days you still find yourself with quite a bit more weight than you had before you conceived, remember that your body needs these reserves to help you through your physical recovery and breast-feeding. Be patient.

If you had a caesarean or received an anaesthesia or

painkiller, you may find that these medical aids have powerful effects on your body and may hamper your appetite. That was what happened to Judith:

> 'Right after the baby was born, I had no appetite. I never do under stress. I ate when they brought me food because I felt like I was losing weight and I wanted to be able to produce milk.'

If you had a strenuous but unmedicated birth, you may find yourself voraciously hungry afterward, especially if you laboured many hours without eating.

This is an exceptional, brief period. It is unlikely to have any extended impact on your eating habits, unless pregnancy and childbirth have some symbolic meaning for you that is related to food. If you found yourself eating a great deal during the pregnancy because you felt you were feeding the baby and being a good mother, now you may find yourself content with less food going into your mouth and more into the baby's. That was Maggie's experience after her caesarean birth:

> 'In the hospital after having the baby, I felt like I was in detox for poisoning myself with junk food for all those months. The first day I didn't want to eat at all. The next day I went on a liquid diet and had two more days of light foods. When I got home, I found I wanted to keep on eating the same way–just things that were bland and light and simple. I had no appetite for the

first six weeks. Some of it was that I was slightly depressed, but I also thought, maybe some people eat like this all the time. It was a new idea for me. I was preoccupied with the baby and hardly thought about myself, much less craved food.'

During your pregnancy, your placenta had been producing oestrogen and progesterone. Now that you no longer have a placenta, the level of these hormones drops radically, which influences many of the remarkable changes that are going on for you, including the change in your uterus. During pregnancy, your breasts prepared themselves for breast-feeding. The placenta had produced a hormone that inhibited actual lactation, but now that is gone, your milk will come in. Meanwhile, your body has increased production of hormones, which are not only involved in milk production but also keep your muscles soft and encourage the creation of fatty tissues. These hormones seem to be nature's way of keeping you cuddly for your baby.

The interaction between hormones and your body changes is complex. We do know that a sudden drop in oestrogen is often accompanied by some physical symptoms, such as sweating (which may leave you drenched in the night), fatigue, heart palpitations, or dizziness. For some women, these are very mild and hardly noticeable; for others, they seem to dominate life for a few days. Similarly, some women are emotionally vulnerable and weepy. Their moods are probably related to the hormonal changes.

Since your body is in such chemical turmoil, we recommend that you treat it with great care. We have found that postnatal women benefit greatly from resting and from eating well. We know how hard it is to take good care of yourself when the demands of the baby seem to be overwhelming, when your whole life has changed and you are recovering from childbirth, but the results are well worth it.

Sue, a professional dancer, describes her predicament, common to many women:

'I felt I'd been through the biggest workout of my life and now I was taking care of my baby. I'd go to the bathroom and realise I was still an invalid and had to do so much to take care of my own physical needs for recuperation, but here I was with this screaming creature that was only twenty-one inches (53 cm) long but dominating my life!

'All of a sudden I envied the friends I'd pooh-poohed before, the ones who hired help for the first few weeks. I would have called an agency that day, but we live in a studio apartment and wouldn't have had room for help. My husband took care of the baby a lot those first days while he stayed home from work, but he didn't know how to help me with the care of my body.

'When friends called asking how we were, we asked them to bring over a meal for us. I never dreamed we'd need so much help!'

The most important preparation you can make during pregnancy is to plan ahead for meals that can be served to you without effort. One solution is to cook in advance and freeze the meals for easy heating later. The other solution is to line up a few close friends or family members who will stop by with a hot meal but not necessarily stay to socialise.

You are probably wondering whether there are special vitamins and nutrients that you need during these particularly stressful days. Nature expects you to use stored energy after childbirth. You and the baby may both want to sleep most of the time. Nevertheless, there are some special nutritional considerations.

Since you have lost blood and amniotic fluid at the birth and will continue to lose blood and fluid through the lochia, you will need both water and iron to prevent deficiencies. As long as you have been careful to drink plenty of water and to have an iron-rich diet through the pregnancy, you should be free from too much concern now. Be careful to get all the vitamins that help your body respond to stress; these include vitamin B_6 (which is in whole grains, beans, and meat), and folic acid (part of the B vitamins and found in liver, fruits, cereal, and eggs). You will want plenty of vitamin C, which helps heal wounds and is in citric fruits, grapes, and many other fruits. Vitamin C is not stored in your body, so you need it daily. Vitamin K is given by injection at most hospitals to encourage blood coagulation and prevent haemorrhaging, so you do not have to worry about getting this in your early postnatal diet. Calcium will continue to be an important nutrient after the birth, especially if you are breast-feeding your baby. As always, you need a wide array of trace elements, the myriad of nutrients that occur in small amounts in fresh foods and whose exact functions in our bodies are not yet understood.

A health practitioner at the hospital should discuss diet with you, though you may be too preoccupied with the baby and with your own recovery to pay much attention. You can meet with a nutritionist later, when you have become more used to your new life. Now, even more than usual, you should avoid empty calories, non-nutritious junk food, and fatty foods.

You may still be taking the same prenatal vitamin and mineral supplement that your doctor or midwife recommended during pregnancy. If it was designed to complement the nutrients that you typically consume in your regular diet, you should continue to do well.

As we said earlier, you are going through rapid hormonal changes. During such times (which many women experience premenstrually), it is helpful to have five or six small meals–little more than snacks–per day rather than three larger ones. You may find it easy to be 'good' during these five days, because you will not be getting out much and other people may be preparing meals for you. If you have no one in the family who can cook for you, we hope that you have stored simple, nutritious food in the freezer. A microwave can be a big help in this period. As important as it is to eat well, it is even more important to get plenty of rest in the first days.

At the end of the first five days, the immediate recovery

period from childbirth, you may look as though you are about seven months pregnant, because your two sets of abdominal muscles separated down the middle, stretched to accommodate the growth of the baby (see below) and have not yet returned to normal. When you lie on your back, your abdomen will not be the mountain that it used to be, and you will not have the vigorous kicking and pressure of the child within, but when you stand up, your stretched muscles and skin will bulge. Both of us have had the devastating experience of hearing the question 'When is your baby coming?' more than a week after we had already given birth.

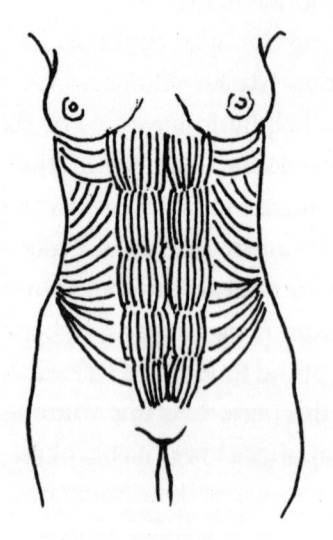

Abdominal muscles pre-pregnancy

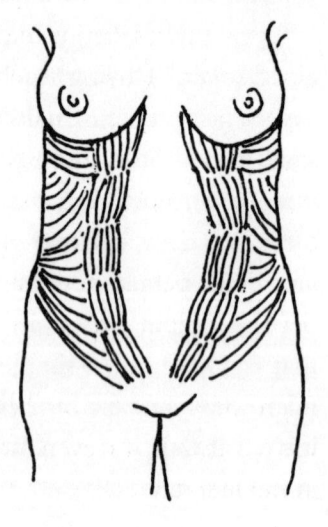

Abdominal muscles in pregnancy

The First Five Days

You almost certainly will not be able to fit into your pre-pregnancy clothes for a while. Maternity outfits will be the most comfortable, but, on principle, you may not want to wear them now. Sensible as it might be to use them, we hear many women say, 'Oh, no, I'm sick of them!' You will find it useful to have several loose-fitting tops that open down the front if you are breast-feeding. With practice, you will find that roomy T-shirts work well also, because you can simply lift up one side and hold the baby to your breast. We recommend that you try to groom yourself to look well and adjust to your newly postnatal figure rather than being disappointed if you cannot get into your familiar clothes.

Mary was speaking for many women when she said:

'Coming home from the hospital the third day after I had my baby, I weighed myself and had lost (9.5 kg) 1½ stone, so I was surprised that I could only wear nightgowns and my maternity clothes. After six weeks or so, the weight just started falling off, but I was shocked in the early period. My breasts were obviously very different and also my stomach and my thighs. I didn't know it was temporary and I was scared!'

You may wonder whether you'll ever feel like yourself again. Perhaps you *are* different now that you have a child. Certainly you will eventually feel more like your pre-pregnancy self than you do now, in the immediate postnatal period. How long it takes depends on many things, such as the temperament of your baby and how much your life has changed. If you return to work quickly, you may find that it does not take very long to settle into your old routine when you are away from home, but then some women feel so profoundly connected to their children that it seems the postnatal period extends until adolescence or beyond! We are dealing with a social and psychological phenomenon as much as the physiological side effect of giving birth.

Don't expect too much from yourself. Observe the wisdom of your baby, who is spending most of his or her time eating and sleeping. Someday both of you will be far more active in the world than you can be this week.

Fatigue is one of the greatest problems of this time. It can result from too little sleep, inadequate diet, too many visitors, or all three. Now is a time for rest and recovery, so pamper yourself.

To help your body heal, start very moderate and isometric exercises the day after giving birth. Obviously, you should NOT be doing an aerobic routine, even if you were in exceptional athletic condition before the birth. The exercises for the first five postnatal days are designed to keep your circulation up and prevent the problems associated with extended bed rest. Remember, women used to call this period the 'confinement' because their activities were so restricted. You must find a happy balance between getting plenty of rest and staying active without straining your system. Your body is vulnerable, so be careful. Here is a good exercise regime for mothers who have had a vaginal delivery.

The First Five Days

The exercises are not suitable after a caesarean birth:

THE BIRTH DAY:

Labour and childbirth are enough exertion for one day!

DAY 1:

Lie on your tummy; place a pillow below your breasts so that you do not put any unnecessary pressure on them (see below).

Lie on your back, bend your knees, feet firmly on bed, and do your Kegel exercises (page 46) – tightening and relaxing your urinary passage, vaginal muscle, and back passage. You won't feel like doing them, as the whole pelvic floor area will be very sore and swollen. But try to persevere, even if you feel you can only tighten your sphincter muscles a little, as this exercise will speed the healing of your episiotomy and subsequently diminish pain and soreness in the area.

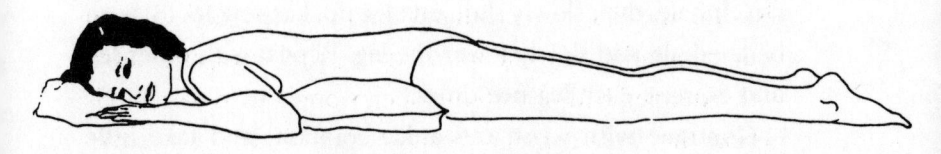

Pillow under tummy

Continue lying on your back, knees bent, and tighten your abdominal muscles–then relax. Repeat this five times.

relaxed   tightened

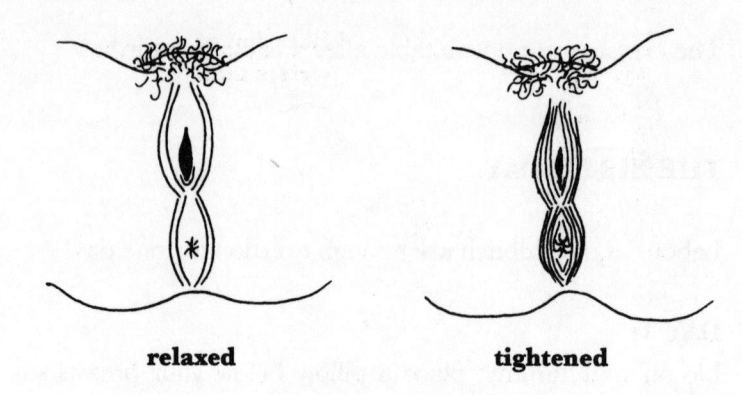

KEGEL EXERCISES

Sit up and rotate your wrists and ankles to increase the circulation and keep your muscles well oiled (page 47).

DAY 2:
Lie on your stomach anytime you feel like it. Repeat the Kegel exercises. Tighten your pelvic floor muscles 3–5 times, twice to three times a day.

Repeat the tightening of the abdominal muscles exercise from day 1.

Add: leg slides (page 47). Lie on your back, legs stretched out. Inhale, then slowly slide one leg up, keeping foot flat on bed, exhale and slowly lower the leg. Repeat with other leg and exercise each leg five times.

Continue with wrist and ankle rotation, and take little walks, watching your posture carefully.

DAY 3:
Repeat lying on your stomach, Kegel exercises, tightening of

The First Five Days

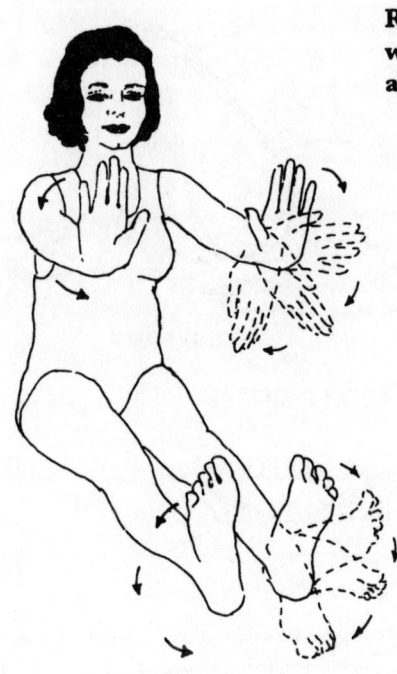

Rotation of wrists and ankles

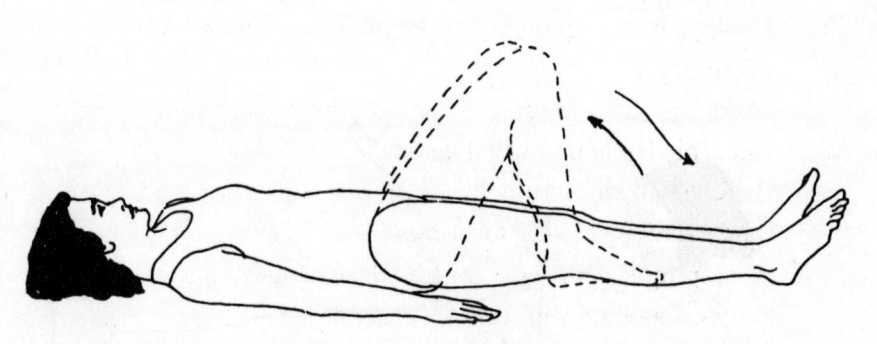

Leg slide

Losing Weight After Pregnancy

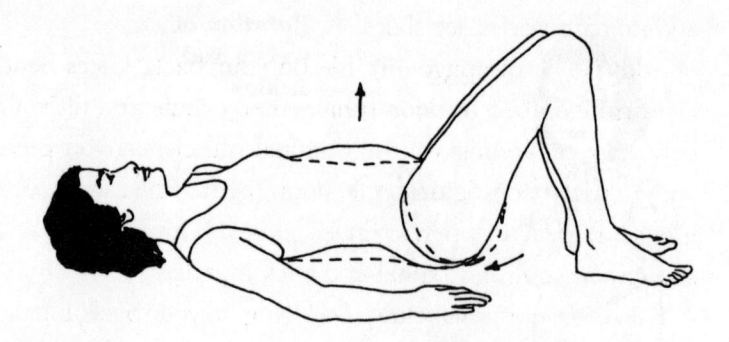

Pelvic tilt

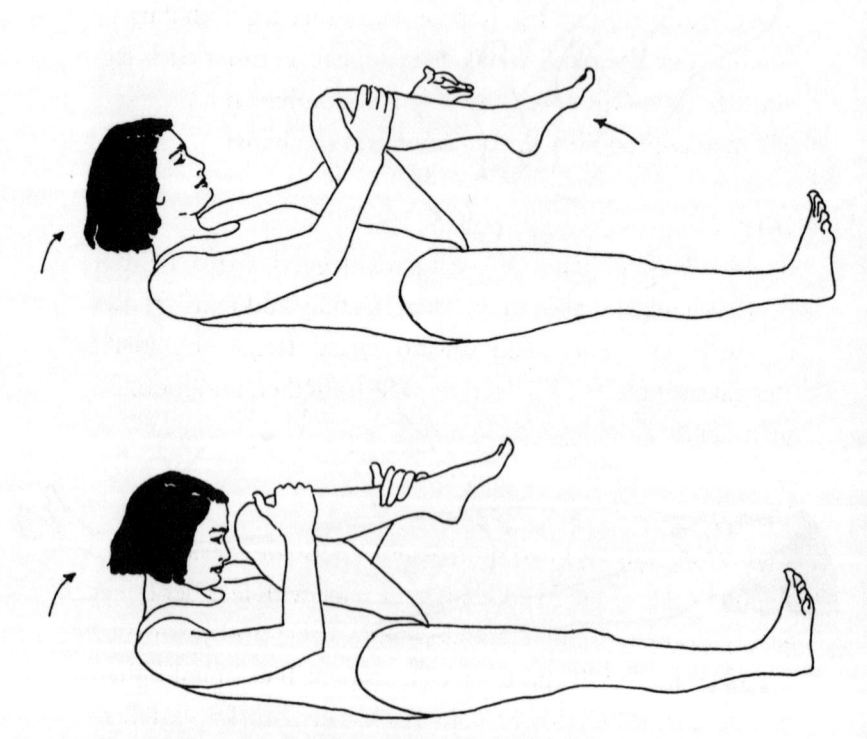

Knee lifts with raising of head

The First Five Days

abdominal muscles, leg slides.

Add: pelvic tilt (page 48). Lie on your back, knees bent, feet firmly on bed or floor. Inhale–then exhale and tilt your pelvis up, tightening your abdominal muscles as you press your lower back against the floor (bed). Release as you inhale. Repeat the pelvic tilt six times. This exercise will strengthen your abdominal and back muscles.

Knee lifts (opposite below). Still lying on your back, inhale, then exhale as you raise one knee toward your chest, at the same time lifting your head toward your knee. Inhale, and lower your head and leg. Repeat with other leg. Exhaling as you lift your knee and your head. Repeat six times each leg. This exercise will strengthen your abdominal muscles and will increase mobility in your knee and hip joints.

DAY 4:

Spinal exercise (page 50). Sit cross-legged, arms behind head, inhale, and arch upper back. Exhale and relax elbows forward and bend head toward chest. Relax shoulders. Repeat five times. This exercise will strengthen and mobilise your spine.

DAY 5:

Today you can add two more exercises to your series.

1 The bridge (page 51). Lie on your back with legs bent, feet firmly on floor or bed. Inhale, then exhale and raise your buttocks slowly off the floor to a straight line. Inhale, then exhale and slowly lower your back, vertebra by vertebra. This exercise will give mobility to your spine and strengthen

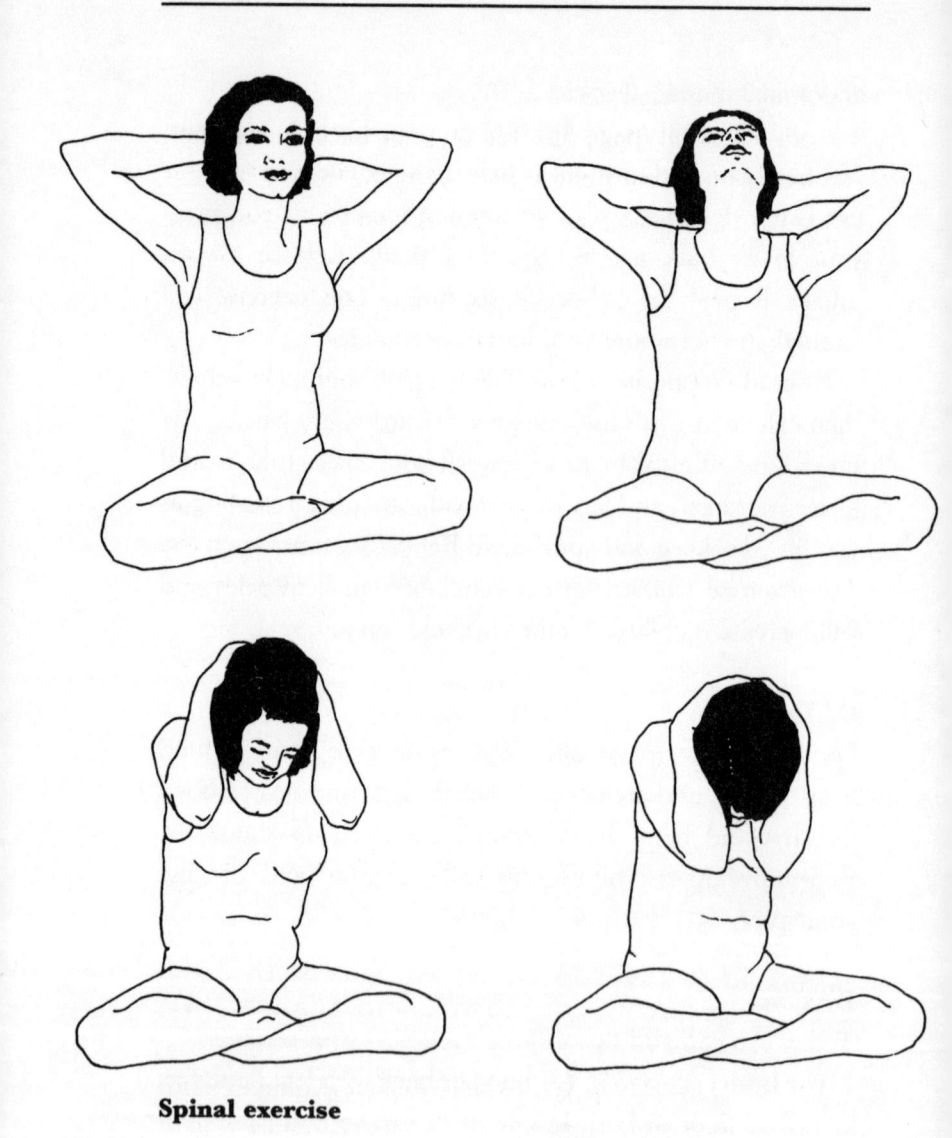

Spinal exercise

abdominal and back muscles. Repeat three times.

2 Modified sit-up (page 52). Lie on your back, knees bent, arms crossed on your chest; inhale, then exhale and raise head and shoulders off the floor. Inhale and lower your head

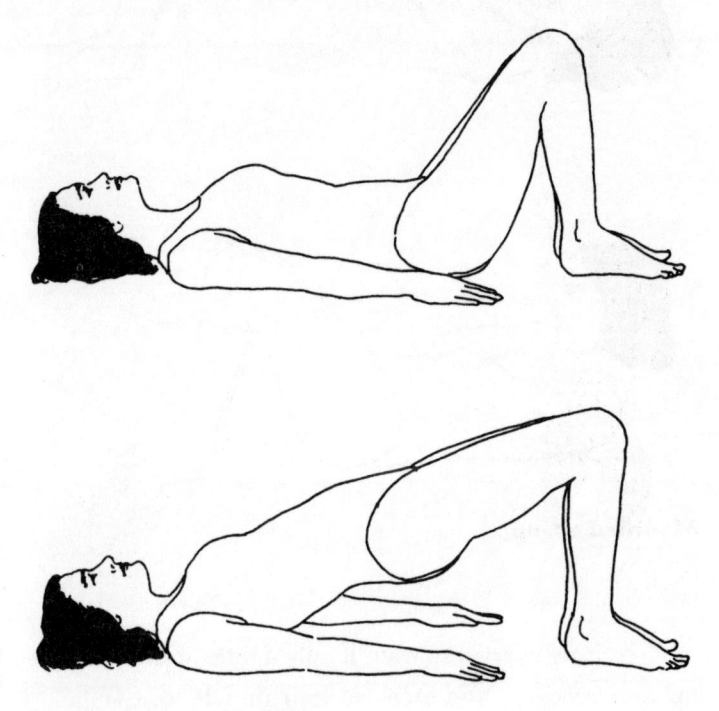

The bridge

and shoulders slowly as you exhale. Repeat five times. This is not an easy exercise, and you should do it carefully, watching that your abdominal muscles will not pop up while you raise your head. It will strengthen your abdominal muscles.

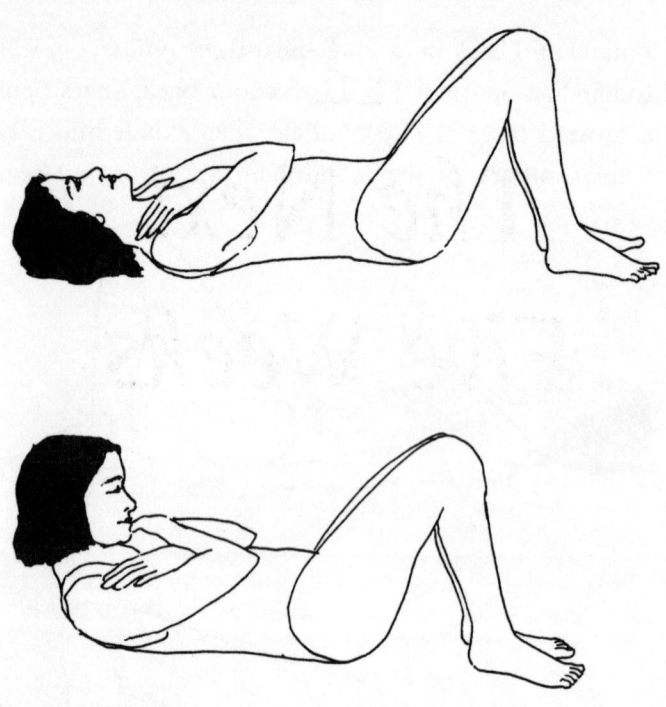

Modified sit-up

Exercising every day, even if only a little at first, will speed up your recovery and increase your muscle tone.

3
The Next Five Weeks

The medical profession has chosen to examine women at six weeks after childbirth because their bodies have generally reached a level of physiological stability by then. We cannot be sure how long it will take for your body to return to normal because there is so much individual variation, but by somewhere around the six-week mark, you should start to feel more like your old self.

The weeks between the first five days and the six-week checkup are still part of a recovery process. During this month, you are still going through many physical changes. This is the period during which your milk supply is established and your uterus heals.

After nine months of gradual changes to provide for the baby, it may take nine months for your body to achieve its pre-pregnancy condition. For instance, as mentioned earlier, the area of the uterus where the placenta had been attached is still in the process of healing. Your body is dealing with the extensive changes of pregnancy and still doing the work of returning to what you consider your normal body. You can expect slight bleeding (lochia) for four weeks or so; it will be full-flowing in the early days – even stronger than a period – but will gradually diminish. The red colour will change to yellowish white and will finally seem like a mucous discharge. If you are breast-feeding, the lochia will stop earlier than if you are not, because breast-feeding stimulates the release of oxytocin, a hormone that makes your uterus contract and therefore helps heal the site where the placenta detached itself.

While oxytocin speeds up the rate at which your uterus returns to its pre-pregnant size, nursing does not mean that your figure will come back right away. It is only the healing of the uterus that is accelerated. To regain a flat belly, you have to allow your muscle and skin tissue to expel the fluid retained during pregnancy and regain their original size and elasticity, a process that may take anywhere from several weeks to several months. To rebuild the tone in your abdominal muscles, you will have to pay special attention to the exercise in your daily routine that uses them most, the modified sit-ups. Be careful to build up your strength slowly.

In these early weeks, you are still working out a routine with your baby and becoming organised enough to be able to pack up your nappy bag, wrestle with the pram, and get yourself out for a trip to the supermarket. You may think that you are the only new mum who doesn't have her baby on a schedule by the time it is six weeks old, but relax. In fact, the majority of babies are still waking several times in the night and still eating and napping without a sense of schedule. Your baby is still learning about the diurnal rhythms of civilisation. While he may be quite regular already, he is perfectly normal if he is not yet eating and napping as you had imagined. Keep working on shaping him to a daily pattern that suits your life-style. Children do benefit from a predictable day, and so do their parents.

A few women are at their happiest when they are caring for a newborn, but most of you will find that it is a period of confusion and frustration, even though it is also joyous and magical. This paradox, the simultaneous presence of conflicting feelings of selfless love and selfish frustration, creates anxiety, which can lead to problems with eating. You may react to the stress by forgetting to eat altogether, which can lead to difficulties with breast-feeding, or by snacking all the time, especially on your favourite comfort foods, which for most of us tend to be things like chocolates and crisps.

You will have to realise that there are such things as empty calories. Symbolically, they are like the love of an exhausted mother. A doughnut *looks* like a lot of food. It fills your stomach. It carries a lot of calories. But it does not give you what you need. Similarly, when you are exhausted and frazzled, you may *look* as if you are doing everything possible for your baby, but you are not able to transfer a sense of profound security and love to her.

Do not go on a radical weight-loss diet yet, whether you are breast-feeding or not. During these first six weeks, your body is still going through complicated physiological adjustments, which are stressful for your metabolism. It is more important to stay healthy and energetic than to regain your pre-pregnancy figure right away, and furthermore you are very likely to continue to lose weight at a surprising rate without even trying.

Several women have said to us, 'If I'm not on a diet, I'll

just gain lots of weight. I can't possibly wait until I stop breast-feeding to go on a diet'. All the women who said this to us were women who had consciously controlled their eating all their adult lives. By the word 'diet', we believe that they meant something quite different from what doctors intend when they tell you not to diet while breast-feeding. When the doctor said 'Don't diet,' she did not mean 'Eat whatever you want whenever you want and grow as fat as you please because it doesn't matter.' She probably meant 'Do not crash-diet' or 'Do not starve yourself.'

We looked up the word 'diet' in *The Concise Oxford Dictionary*, which confirmed that it does have two quite different meanings. On the one hand, it refers to 'way of feeding' or to 'one's habitual food'; on the other hand, it means 'special food as medical regimen or punishment'. When doctors tell women not to diet during pregnancy or while breast-feeding, they mean that you should not restrict yourself to a regime that would deprive you of the calories and nutrients you need to keep yourself and your developing baby strong and healthy. But taken in another sense, postnatal women should be very aware of their diet—not for weight loss or punishment, but for energy and for building a healthy baby and a healthy mother.

Ideally, all nutrients should come through a good diet of fresh, natural foods, including plenty of fruits and vegetables, but just now your priority is to keep life simple and your energy high. Jane shared her worries about eating:

'I have the feeling that there are so many things I am

supposed to be getting, you know, calcium, vitamins, minerals, and if I eat enough to get everything that I need, I will put on lots of weight.'

Relax and just try to eat as wide a variety of foods as you can manage, but do not stuff yourself. A newborn does not eat very much. If you are breast-feeding, you will be burning extra calories in the process of creating milk and supplying the calories that are in the milk itself. For now, you probably use about 500 calories for breast-feeding. If your baby is exclusively breast-fed at six months, you may expend 1,000 or more calories in the milk itself and in the process of creating it. If you eat 2,500 nutritious calories a day while breast-feeding, you will almost surely lose weight gradually over the months.

Your body will make sure that the necessary nutrients get into the milk. The important thing for you is to remember to eat well so that there will be enough essential vitamins and minerals left for your body to stay strong. We know that calcium can be taken from a woman's own bones if she is not consuming enough for milk production. That can lead to osteoporosis, brittle bones that break easily. Now more than ever, you need extra calories *and* good nutrition. Eat not only milk products and fish like sardines that you can eat bones and all, but also eat such potassium-rich goods as bananas, dried apricots, and broccoli, which will help your body metabolise calcium.

You will find that your whole life is disrupted by the baby and that good eating patterns are hard to achieve in the first few weeks. The microwave is a great help, for you can heat up a cup of soup in one minute or bake a potato to top with low-fat yogurt in six minutes. Fresh raw vegetables and cheese will be handy as easy nutritious snacks throughout the day. A banana is always satisfying and takes no preparation at all. Connie admitted:

'Sometimes I don't have a chance to get lunch unless someone else is there to help me make it. I have a woman who comes in the mornings to help with housekeeping. I have started using her to make sure I get nutritious foods to start the day. She fixes yogurt and fruit for me on the days that she is there. My husband usually cooks supper. When I am alone, I grab a piece of cheese when I can't fix a meal. Both my eating and my sleeping patterns have been disrupted in ways that are against my natural rhythms.'

Virginia used what she had learned from her first experience the second time around:

'In the early weeks, I was not sleeping and I was spending all my time getting to know that baby and nursing him. I had trouble keeping up with my own need to eat. It was a real challenge to even eat lunch. When I had my first child, I'd see that it was three o'clock in the afternoon and I hadn't eaten anything. I'd be weak and tired and grouchy. I realised that if I were to survive I had to be sure to eat. Now, with the second baby, I keep carrot sticks and peanut butter, and cans of tuna fish packed in water available all the time.'

Just as the grass is always greener on the other side of the fence, you may feel that all your friends look slender and wonderful immediately after they have their babies, and you wonder, Why don't I? You were probably not looking at their bodies as carefully as you look at your own. Rachel talks about that problem:

'I was with a good friend two weeks after she had her baby and I asked, 'Where is your tummy? It looks so flat!' She pulled up her shirt and took hold of the loose skin over her belly and I realised that to her it seemed very different, but from the outside it looked fine. Now that it is two weeks since I gave birth, I remember her belly, and mine looks similar. That's how I realised that it is simply the way things are for now. I find it rather interesting to watch my body go through such profound changes. It isn't only in my belly, but also on my hips and thighs. Now I'm watching my body getting back into form. It is absolutely fascinating, just to watch it every day and see what shape it is in now. When I take my bath, I press my tummy and see how far below the waterline it goes now. I can see the difference day by day.'

One of the mothers we interviewed said, 'My baby is three weeks old and I have been totally absorbed in her, but all of a sudden I have this incredible urge to go out again with my husband. Am I a bad mother if I leave my baby with a sitter so soon?' We feel that any impulse toward self-renewal shows you are emerging from the early days and re-engaging in life outside. If you provide good enough substitute care, you will be taking care of yourself and the baby by having fun. You may be a new mother, but you are also a person with other interests.

One of the great advantages of having other familiar caregivers for the baby is that no one person will burn out or get overburdened. If you have a regular sitter (preferably a friend or family member who will be part of the baby's life forever), you will be freer to love your baby joyously when you are with her. You will not get as fatigued and you will not feel as deprived. Just as your diet of food should be varied and complex, so your diet of activities needs variety for greater emotional health.

The ability to ask for and accept help is one of the best psychological traits that we know of. Every study of childbearing women shows that the mothers who do best are the ones who say they have loving help at home, especially the caring support of their partner. Even researchers who expected to find that the most competent mothers were the ones who scored highest on scales of self-reliance found the opposite. Mothers who reported that they received the most support seemed to be the least depressed.

It is especially important for caregivers to avoid martyrdom. We can get so dedicated to our fantasy of 'good mother' that we stress ourselves beyond our limit of endurance. A good mother makes sure that her baby is always getting loving care. The mother herself cannot provide that care if she is too exhausted to stand.

Here are ten practical suggestions for living your life in a way that will help you stay healthy and watch your weight gradually drop away even during this period of stress and change:

1. Eat when you are hungry but before you get too hungry. As we suggested for the first five days, since you probably do not have time or energy to eat large, regular meals, we recommend that you take smaller, easier meals more times a day. Just as your baby is eating frequently, so too will you benefit from small, nutritious snacks that do not overwhelm your system.

You may be worried that all these snacks will make it harder to get back to your pre-pregnancy weight. We urge you to be patient. You are still in the very early weeks and will have plenty of time to address your figure after the dramatic physiological changes have stabilised. You will probably find that if you can stay relaxed (no easy feat!) and content with the complicated task of managing your baby and adjusting to your new life-style, and if you stay away from empty calories such as those obtained through sugar or alcohol (lot of calories but very little nutrition), 20–25 pounds will have melted away by your six-week checkup.

2. Learn to love whole-grain breads and cereals. They are a rich source of complex carbohydrates and contain B vitamins that are often deficient in the typical Western diet. They are also a good source of fibre. Brewer's yeast is an especially rich source of B vitamins and many trace elements whose exact purposes aren't yet understood.

While it is always a good idea to add a new wholesome item to your diet, we think you will have the most success if you create your healthy diet by changing from non-nutritious food to nutritious versions of the same food, rather than by altering your life-style. You want to make changes that will last, not to be distracted by gimmicks. You have always eaten bread; simply change from white to whole wheat. You have always eaten rice. Now, prepare brown rice rather than polished rice. Switch from jam or marmalade to whole-fruit spread. If you drink whole milk, switch to semi-skimmed. If you already drink semi-skimmed switch to skimmed.

In general, choose the same foods as usual, but buy them in their unprocessed forms so that you can benefit from all the nutrients that they contain. Eat everything, especially fruits and vegetables, as fresh as possible.

3. Learn to tolerate liver and spinach. An iron-poor diet (not unusual, even among affluent Western women) leads to iron-deficiency anaemia, which results in fatigue and listlessness. As long as you are losing red blood cells through lochia, you need to boost your iron intake and be sure that you get plenty of vitamins C and E, which help with iron absorption.

Liver and spinach are not the only sources of iron. Meat, eggs (especially the yolk), whole-grain breads, cereals, and wheat germ are also iron-rich. Blackstrap molasses is another readily available item, which tastes reasonably good and is rich in iron. You can add a tablespoon to a cup of skimmed milk and heat it in the microwave for a delicious and nutritious substitute for coffee.

4. Eat a salad with at least three different vegetables in it at least once a day. A wide variety of foods will supply a wide variety of nutrients. You may not have the time or interest to choose exactly what food will satisfy what nutritional requirement each day, so the easiest thing to do is just to make sure you eat lots of different things. All fresh vegetables are good for you, not only for nutrients but also for fibre, which keeps your intestines functioning well.

Get a large plastic bowl with a tight-fitting lid. Wash a batch of greens, dry them, tear them into salad-size pieces, and keep them in the bowl along with carrots and celery so that you have the basis of your salad ready at all times.

Be creative! You can put fruit as well as vegetables in your salads. Make sure your vegetables come in lots of different colours, which may indicate they are from different families and therefore will supply different nutrients.

Now that supermarkets are packaging pre-washed greens and pre-chopped vegetables, it is easier than ever to toss together a great salad. Try a combination of spinach leaves, apple chunks, sunflower seeds, and raisins, tossed with a little bit of lemon juice. You won't need any other dressing and you will be consuming a delightful variety of nutrients. Take a glass of non-fat milk and a slice of whole-grain bread along with it and you have a perfect small meal.

5. Remember to drink plenty of fluids. Actually, your body should remind you of this. You will probably feel thirsty enough to consume at least two quarts of fluids a day–to replace what you are losing through discharge and breast-feeding.

You don't have to drink milk to produce milk. Count on your mammary glands to create the milk, and feel free to drink water and juice while making sure you get plenty of calcium through a variety of dairy products. If you are allergic to milk, you can still breast-feed as long as you get the necessary calcium through non-dairy sources, such as sardines and canned salmon or a supplement recommended by your health-care provider.

Many women find that shakes are the handiest way to get nutrition and fluids in an easily created and easily consumed form. You can start with non-fat yogurt, milk, or juice and add any fruit you wish, along with some ice cubes, and run them in the blender. Bananas are particularly handy for shakes. Frozen berries work well also.

6. Eat plenty of protein in the form of fish, poultry, and lean meats. You need the protein for your own body and for milk production if you are breast-feeding. The typical American diet includes a lot of protein from red meats, but we caution you against getting all of it in this form because red meats are laced with more animal fat than you need. When we eat fat, we readily convert it to fat, which gets stored in our bodies. You want to avoid that. Instead, consume complex carbohydrates or proteins that come without animal fats.

7. Avoid sugar, salty foods, alcohol and nicotine. They do not contribute any nutrients and have an adverse affect on your health, especially if consumed in large quantities. In fact, many diets begin by suggesting as complete an elimination of sugar as you can achieve. Sugar tastes great, but you don't need it. Now that you are on call around the clock for your baby, you do need to keep your body as balanced as possible. Fuel it with a steady diet of healthy foods, not the quick fix of a sugar rush.

Salt exaggerates the natural tendency of your body to retain water. If you don't want that puffy look, keep your salt intake down. That means avoiding the flavour enhancer monosodiumglutamate (MSG) as well. Stick with fresh foods that carry their own natural flavours instead of items prepared with additives that trick your brain into thinking you've eaten something good.

8. Be sure to rest whenever your baby sleeps during the day, as long as your sleep is being interrupted during the night. Take the telephone off the hook and put a 'Do Not Disturb' sign on your door if necessary. Rest may do more than extra calories to help you keep up your energy. Your health and well-being are influenced by more than simply what and how you eat. To regain your figure and control your eating habits, you must be relaxed and happy.

9. Ask for help when you feel stressed. Even if you are very sensible in your eating and sleeping patterns, you may find that you occasionally get driven to distraction by the demands of your baby. If you do not have anyone who can take over with the baby, pack him in your baby carrier and go for a walk. If it is pouring or you are too tired to walk, take him for a drive in the car. Your baby will almost certainly fall asleep the moment you drive away. Don't forget that there are parenting organisations that can offer support (see page 136). Anytime that you feel you are inadequate or you are afraid you might lose your temper, call their hot lines or call your GP or call a friend. Do not let yourself become isolated. Too many of us turn to food when we are stressed. Turn toward help instead.

10. Watch out for being too sedentary. Just because you can't return to a rigorous programme at the gym doesn't mean that you cannot get out and walk! We have found that many of the women whose bodies recover from childbirth most quickly are those who were exercising regularly before they became pregnant and continued to exercise sensibly through the pregnancy.

Pay attention to your own body to determine how strenuous you should be. For example, if you are walking with a friend, choose a pace slow enough so that you can still carry on a conversation but brisk enough for it to have some effect when you are talking. In these early weeks, it is lovely to have your baby in the sling so that you can chat with him while you walk. You don't need to run a marathon or climb a mountain to establish a good pattern of exercise. A relaxed stroll that lasts an hour will elevate your metabolism and burn up calories of stored fat but won't stress you at all. A walk before a meal will get your body ready to burn up the calories you eat. A gentle walk after a meal will stimulate your stomach to digest your food more rapidly

Make sure you walk in the most enjoyable places you can think of. The more you enjoy your outings, the more you will look forward to them and fit them into your life. You are trying to establish a pattern of regular exercise that will last the rest of your life. Make it realistic and make it fun!

Exercise will increase your metabolism and help you burn up extra calories. See if you can find a postnatal exercise class with a baby-sitter. They are available in many communities, and not only help you get your figure back but also prevent social isolation.

Many women want to get back to the gym as soon as possible. If you do resume exercise during the first four to five weeks, be sure it is with the approval of your doctor and under the supervision of a person who knows about postnatal recovery. Remember, from the outside you might look perfectly normal. The instructor cannot see your vulnerable uterus or understand the metabolic changes going on unless you tell her.

Check with your doctor or nurse-midwife before taking on any new or vigorous exercise programme. Start slowly and pay attention to how it feels. Women who work out strenuously are at risk from bleeding and hampering their healthy recovery from childbirth. Be particularly careful of your abdominal muscles and those of your pelvic floor.

We know quite a few women who teach prenatal and postnatal exercise classes. All of them stay very fit and regain excellent abdominal tone within weeks of having a baby, but not within days. And they do not resume teaching right away. As professionals in the field of exercise (and some of them are professional dancers), they know how to read the internal signals of their bodies and are careful not to overdo it. Here is the account of a teacher of prenatal and postnatal exercises:

'The first time I returned to exercise class after my daughter was born, it was as a student, not as a teacher. I was very excited about it. I expressed some milk in advance and gave the bottle to the child-care worker. I felt sure there was no need of hers that couldn't be taken care of, so I allowed myself to focus fully on myself for an hour, and it was wonderful! The stretching and breathing were grand. I was in heaven, just breathing and not worrying about her for a whole hour!

'I don't feel ready to teach again yet. I feel I keep coming back to myself in stages and I haven't created that balance in myself yet. I'm giving out so much mothering I don't want to mother anybody else yet. I need more time before I start adding taking care of other people as well. It would still deplete more than nurture me.'

Sandy told us how she dealt with her desire for exercise without using child care:

'I did abdominal exercises regularly from the beginning of pregnancy and walked two or three miles a day. Although I gained 2 stone 10 pounds (17.2 kg), I had no stretch marks. I was pretty shaky at first. The day after I got home from the hospital, I just walked round the block and back. Then I tried to go a little further each day. I took our first trip to a museum two weeks after giving birth. Now I go out every day with her in the sling. In a couple of months I'll switch to the pram. I'll use any excuse: errands, museums, lunch with friends, to see her father at work. I'll invent an errand thirty minutes away just to get the exercise.'

Remember the importance of establishing a regular routine of exercise so that it becomes a natural part of your life. Once a week isn't enough. Studies show that a healthy person should exercise for at least half an hour at least three times a week. At a sensible level of moderate exercise, every day is even better. If you cannot find it in your schedule to take one long outing a day, see if you can get three or four ten-minute jaunts–to the bank, around the block, anywhere! Take the stairs instead of the escalator whenever you have the chance. In every activity, work toward a vigorous pace that will tone your muscles and slightly elevate your heart rate, just enough to pick up your metabolism and keep you healthy.

Here are the exercises we think are especially well suited for new mothers:

Start with a series that are done lying down (see pages 47–52).

- Kegels
- Rotations
- Leg slides
- Pelvic tilt
- Knee lifts
- Spinal exercise
- The bridge
- Modified sit-ups

Now stand. Do the following.

Roll-down (see pages 73–4).
Stand straight, inhale. Exhale and slowly relax and bend down, relaxing the spine vertebra by vertebra. Then inhale and slowly straighten up to a standing position. Repeat five times. This exercise will give you spinal mobility.

The Next Five Weeks

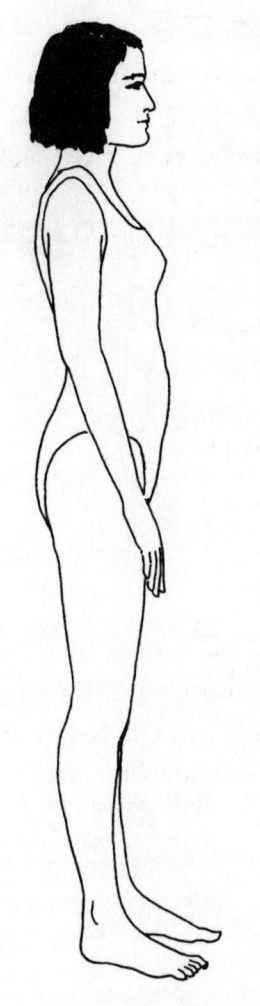

Roll-down No. 1

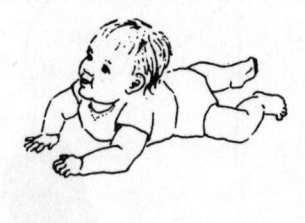

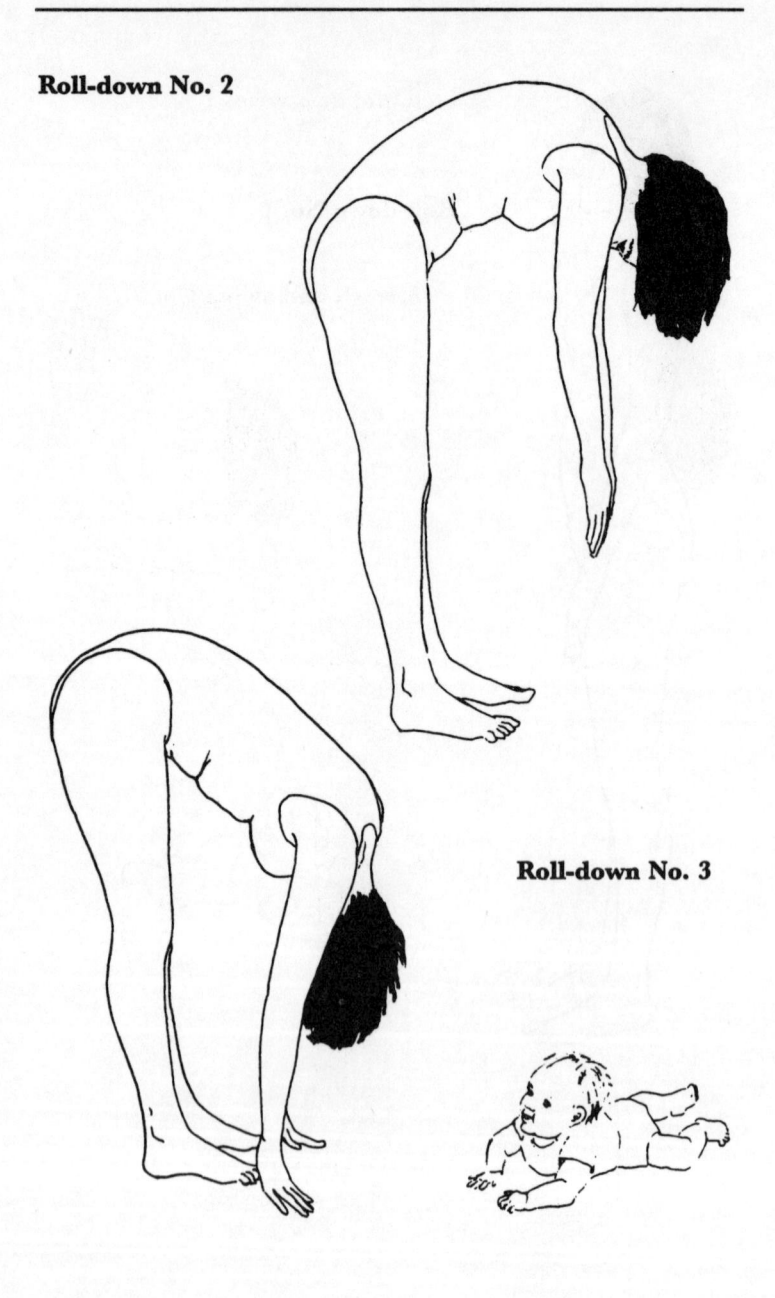

Roll-down No. 2

Roll-down No. 3

Stretch and swing No. 1

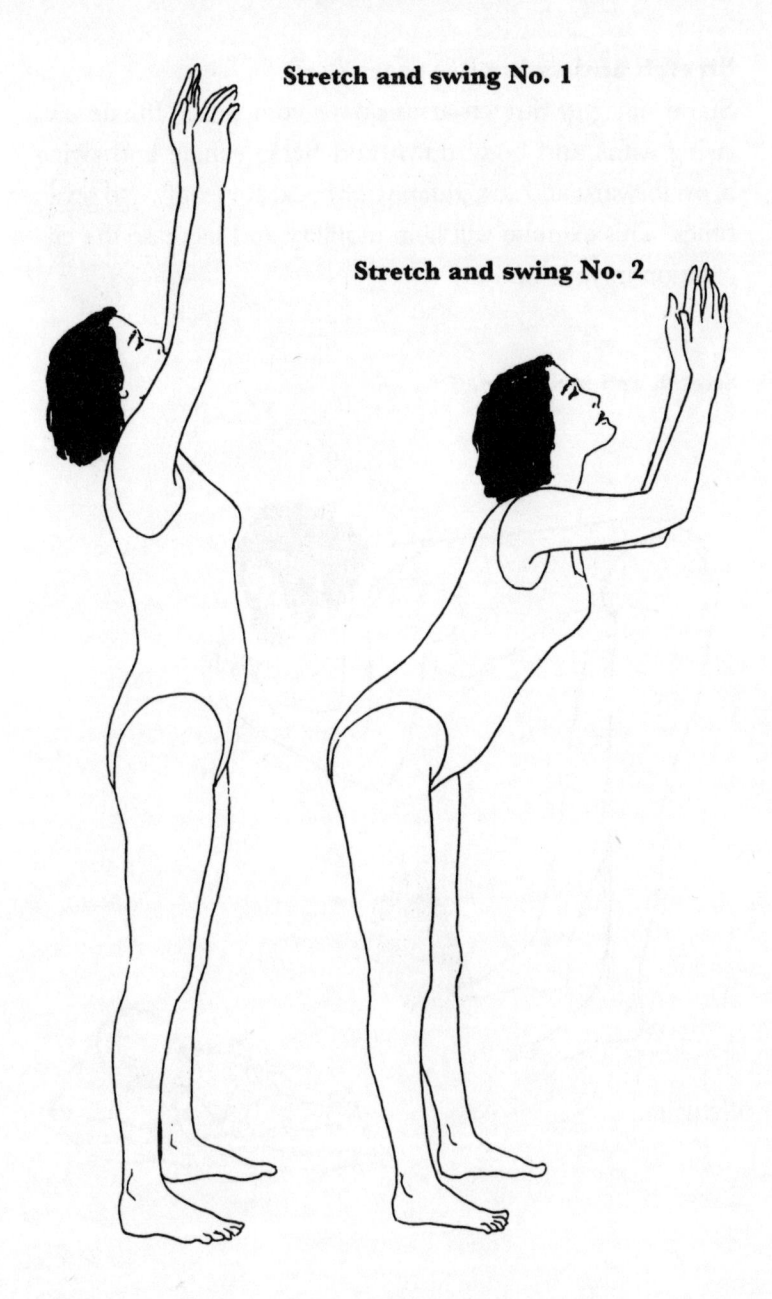

Stretch and swing No. 2

Stretch and swing (see pages 75–7).
Stand upright. Stretch arms above your head. Inhale and swing arms and body down and back, exhale and swing arms forward and straighten your back. Repeat five to seven times. This exercise will help mobility and increase the circulation in your body.

Stretch and swing No. 3

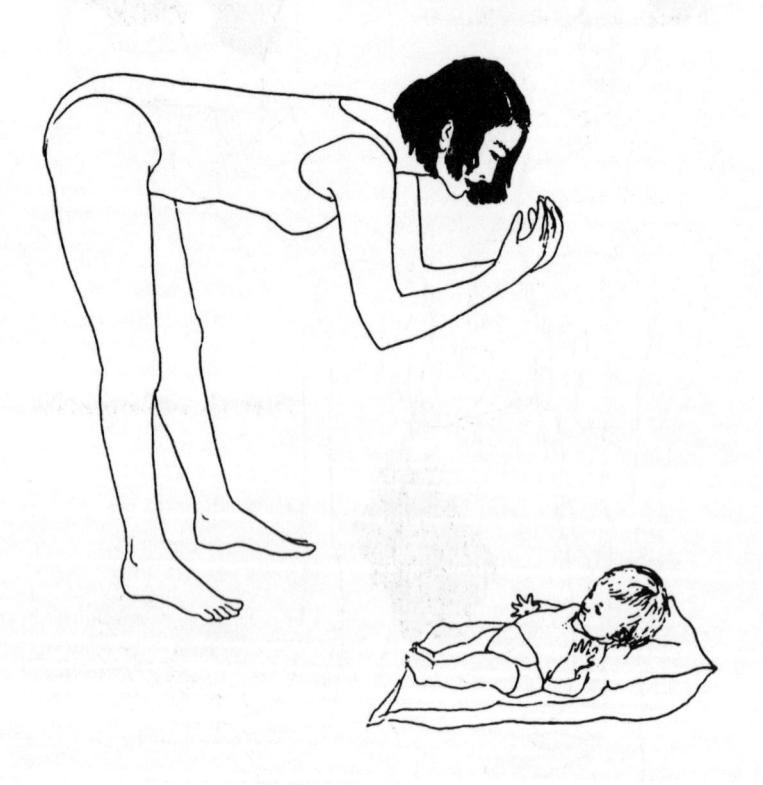

Stretch and swing No. 4

Stretch and swing No. 5

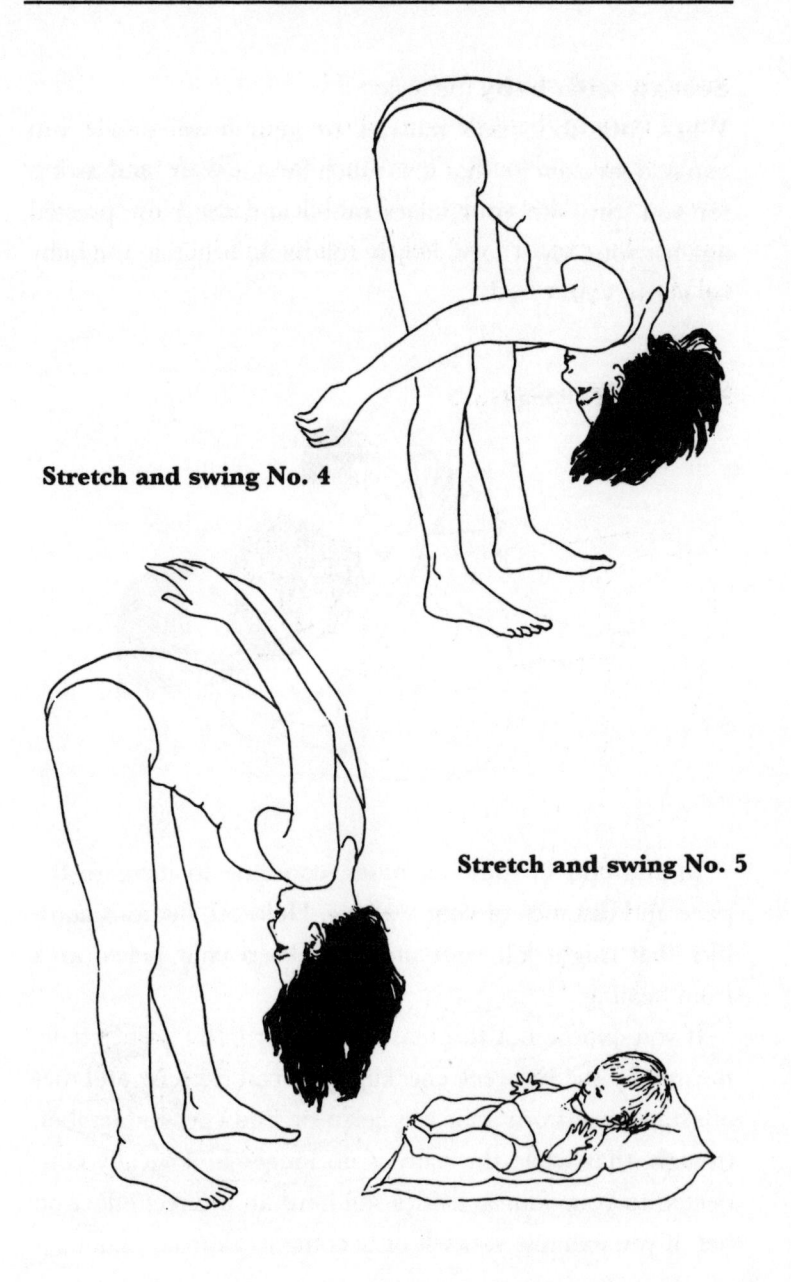

Seesaw with baby (below).
When your abdominal muscles are getting well toned, you can add an exercise that is as much fun for your baby as it is for you. Sit with your knees raised and the baby pressed against your lower legs. Slowly roll back, bringing the baby up above you.

Seesaw with baby

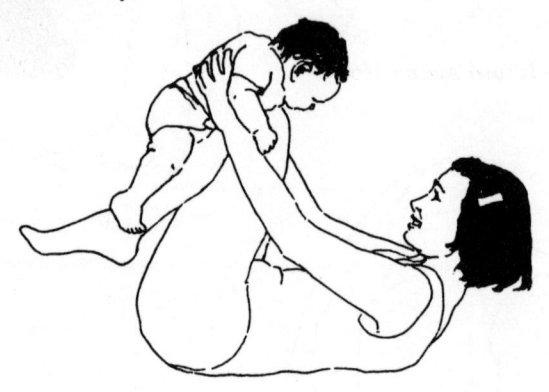

In addition to these exercises, continue to increase the pace and distance of your walking. Hold off vigorous aerobics that might jolt your uterus or keep your pelvic area from healing.

If you choose not to breast-feed, your body is essentially normal by the six-week checkup. You can exercise and diet after an okay from your physician or midwife. Remember, though, that while the baby is no longer biologically connected to you, your activities still have an indirect effect on her. If you exhaust yourself or become weak from malnutrition, you will not be able to have the energy to get up in the night or be patient with the demands of mothering. Even though you have a good bill of health from the doctor, be careful not to try to lose weight too rapidly. This is still a time to take special care of yourself and to be patient with the changes in your figure. Continue with the exercises recommended earlier in the book. Eat well and gradually grow more active.

4

Losing Weight While Breast-Feeding

We have listened to women debate the question of whether they lose more weight while breast-feeding or lose it more easily after they stop. Some swear that they have never lost weight as easily as they did while nursing. Others say they kept the weight on as long as they were breast-feeding and then dropped 7 pounds (about 3.2 kg) or so right after weaning. Who's right?

Both, of course. Some women stay the same weight or even gain while breast-feeding, but most lose 2–4 pounds (0.9–1.8 kg) per month without even trying if they feed their baby exclusively with breast milk for the first four to six months.

As long as you are lactating, your breasts stay large and keep an extra pound or two on your body that will show up on the scale, but because your body is burning up extra calories every day, not only in the milk itself but also in the process of creating it, you should lose weight if you continue to eat at your previous level while you are breast-feeding. You might find that you are eating more than usual or that your metabolism has slowed down and you do not want to lose weight until you have weaned your baby. That is fine, too.

When we think about weight gain or weight loss, most of us think in terms of calories. The word 'calorie' stands for a unit of measurement, but it is an abstract concept, because it does not measure size. Rather, it measures the release of heat or energy. When we talk about how many calories you should consume in a day, it is not at all like talking about how many apples you should eat. A calorie is not a physical object, although we generally talk as though it were.

The usual recommendation is for an average adult woman to consume about 2,000 calories a day, a pregnant woman to have 2,300, and a lactating woman 2,500. What exactly does this mean in terms of your life and your weight? It means that most lactating women release 2,500 calorie units of energy in the course of a typical day. If you are tall and large-boned, you will need more calories than if you are petite. If you have a very fast metabolism, you will release more energy than if you have a very slow metabolism. If you take a brisk three-mile walk, your body will burn up over 200 extra calories in the process. If you are nursing a drowsy newborn, as you can imagine, you don't release as many units of energy feeding him as if you were nursing an active six-month-old who is starting to crawl. Once your baby is eating solid foods, he won't be stimulating you to burn as many calories as he was before.

So when we talk about a lactating woman needing 2,500 calories a day from her food, we are talking about an average. The actual number of calories you burn daily varies a great deal. In general, we think in terms of consuming food that will be capable of releasing about the number of calories that we need for our activities in that day, but remember, you need more than just calories. You need specific nutrients that will help your body perform specific important duties, like keeping your bones strong, your organs functioning, and your skin healthy.

Your metabolism also changes as you age. Quite obviously, a fifteen-year-old can eat enormous amounts and not put on an ounce. When you are still growing, most of the calories you consume in food may be burned just to produce the new cells needed for your growth. Protein is especially important for the creation of new cells, and so it is important as long as you are lactating, for that is a process of creating new cells.

All lactating women need much more calcium than others, and we must point out that a breast-feeding teenager needs enough calcium not only to create the good milk for her baby but also to build her own bones, which are still growing. Once you are fully grown, your body requires fewer calories and you may need more exercise in order to burn the amount of calories that you have got into the habit of eating.

Some women feel voraciously hungry for as long as they are breast-feeding. This may be a product of the increased demand on their energy. If you are physically active and your baby has a big appetite, you will be able to consume a lot of calories without worrying about weight gain. For a few women, the concern is in the other direction. They find that they cannot eat enough to get ahead.

Presumably, well-nourished women can get by with less

fat in reserve because their regular diets are so rich and nutritious, but we were built to store enough fat during pregnancy to be able to sustain a baby for some months after its birth. Lactation naturally follows pregnancy and childbirth. If you do not breast-feed, you disrupt a physiological sequence and may need to adjust accordingly.

We know that female rats that do not suckle their young are more likely to grow obese than those that do. If your body has been storing extra energy in the form of fat during the pregnancy, it is logical that the fat should be intended for fuelling the baby's growth in the six months when (as in pre-industrial times) if would be fully dependent on the breast for sustenance. If you do not breast-feed, you will have to burn off the extra weight in other ways.

As we have said before, the childbearing year is not a time for a radical weight-loss programme that reduces your weight under a healthy level. You are not likely to have the slender figure of a fashion model while you are lactating. The extra fat of the nursing pad will help you feel comfortable to the baby. As one woman put it, 'It is okay for a mother to look cosier.' Another told us that her childbirth educator had asked the class, 'Which would you rather be, a Barbie doll or a koala bear?' Any other year you might choose to be a Barbie doll. For now, consider the virtues of the koala.

In discussing the first six weeks after giving birth, we gave the same advice for those of you who are breast-feeding and those of you who are not. You were in the middle of a powerful physical process and needed to take special care of your body. We told you to get plenty of rest, exercise with care, and eat without trying to lose weight (though pounds probably fell off as your body shed the water retained in pregnancy).

Now the early recovery period is over, but if you are lactating, your body is still quite different from its pre-pregnant state. Most obviously, your breasts are larger. Less visibly, your hormones are in a special state designed to make milk; that is, you are high in progesterone and prolactin production and low in oestrogen production. This new balance will produce some noticeable side effects. For example, you may not resume menstruating for several months. Some women do not ovulate or menstruate as long as they lactate, but don't count on that. Breast-feeding is not a reliable form of birth control. Another of the mysteries of lactation is that is slows down your metabolism and helps you absorb food from your intestines more efficiently.

Nursing changes your life-style as well as your body. It is time-consuming. Your baby may suck for ten minutes and then doze off, but then wake up and suck some more. A meal may take anywhere from half an hour to an hour; sometimes it feels as though you've just finished one feeding when the baby is ready for another, especially in the early weeks. Gradually, your baby will become more organised and be more awake while eating and more interested in other aspects of his life when not eating, but you may be surprised at how much of your life seems dedicated to attending to his needs.

If you are in a rush, nursing will be frustrating for you and your baby. Not everyone is temperamentally suited to it. If you are choosing to be the one to feed the baby, design your day so that you are free to do it well. Your body and your baby will suffer if you are too tired or too tense.

The early weeks and months of parenthood are spent learning how to design your life around a dependent, helpless person while trying not to lose all sense of yourself. Nursing is the epitome of that experience. If you find a way to enjoy the nursing as much as the baby does, you will discover a great opportunity to relax. Set yourself up in a comfortable position with a good pillow supporting you and play your favourite music in the background as you settle in for a good long encounter with your baby. Use the breastfeeding time to catch your breath. The baby is happy eating and you can rest comfortably. You are not getting a full night's sleep, so you need these breaks during the day.

Even though nursing takes up a great deal of your time, you may find it more convenient than the alternative. Preparation of formula and bottle and teat is time-consuming also. The breast is the preferred alternative for many mothers. The milk is always delivered at the right temperature, it is always on tap, and the baby always gets the benefit of being held close to your body during feedings. In addition, breast milk always has the right consistency and, in fact, as your baby grows, your milk changes to keep up with his requirements. After all, human breast milk has evolved to nurture human infants. It provides just what they need for their growth and development.

Many studies have demonstrated the benefits of breast-feeding to the infant; far fewer have focused on the benefits of breast-feeding to the mother. Extended breast-feeding may decrease your risk of breast cancer. Breast-feeding also provides psychological as well as physical benefits for the mother. For example, Julie shared her experience with us:

> 'I wanted to be happy about having a baby, but I couldn't get it together to eat in a way I felt okay about during pregnancy. I had been depressed about my bingeing for nine months, but it all changed as soon as the baby was born. Once she was on the outside and I could see that she was enjoying the breast, I found that I could relax. I just hadn't wanted to deprive her before she was born, so I overate and gained 2 stone 12 pounds (18.1 kg). Now I've settled down.'

Breast-feeding was a learning experience for Julie. She had been nervous throughout the pregnancy, but suddenly she felt like a 'good enough' mum. This is not everyone's experience. Some mothers get nervous because they cannot see how much the baby has eaten. Try to remember that breast-feeding has a built-in wisdom that modulates our tendencies to overfeed or underfeed our children. As Dr. Irwin Chabon, author of *Awake and Aware: Participating in Childbirth Through Psychoprophylaxis,* used to say, 'The annals of medicine have never proven that any baby committed suicide by starving itself. Similarly, an exclusively breast-fed baby is unlikely to become obese. Your regular visits to the baby clinic will reassure you that the baby is developing in a healthy way. You can tell that she is getting enough milk if her nappies are wet and her urine smells normal at expectable intervals.

If you find yourself losing weight while you are breast-feeding, remember that you don't want to become too thin as long as your baby is still dependent on your milk supply for nourishment. The few women we have known who were very thin after giving birth all found themselves exhausted much of the time. They did not have enough energy in reserve to give so many calories a day to the baby and have enough left for themselves.

The most important factor in successful breast-feeding is the general health and nutrition of the mother. You must eat well to produce good milk. Even though your time is filled with infant care, you must remember to take care of yourself as well. Drink plenty of fluids to help make that milk. Water, of course, is an essential ingredient for creating milk and has no calories at all. You need plenty of calcium and protein and all the other important vitamins and minerals that will sustain your health and your baby's as well. If you are concerned about losing weight, be extra careful that the foods you eat are very nutritious but not fattening, so that you can pack all the vitamins and minerals you need into your allotted calories.

Establish a routine of regular nutritious meals and exercise. This may sound like a far-off dream to you when the baby has been demanding all of your attention. As Ellen told us,

> 'One day I found myself still in my nightgown when my husband came home. Where had the day gone? How could I have spent so many hours doing nothing but take care of the baby? Is this me?'

You aren't the perfect mother that you had planned to be. It's been more than six weeks and you may not have a routine yet. Relax. Most babies do not eat at regular times until they are close to four months old. Your job now is to gradually shape the baby to live according to the rhythms that work in your family.

If weight gain and eating patterns have been troublesome issues in your life, assume that they will continue to be at least as troublesome during lactation and may even be compounded by the guilt you feel when you read about things that you 'should' be doing or 'should' be feeling.

As long as you are breast-feeding, you may find that you get exhausted if you skip meals. There are a lot of little tricks you can do to make it through a day when you hardly have a moment to spare. Some women keep sliced cheese to eat when they don't have time to prepare lunch. Others put together a peanut-butter sandwich on whole-grain bread to make sure that they are getting some nutrition with little fuss. Rice cakes and cucumber slices are both handy treats that carry some nutrition. Bananas are old standbys for most nursing mothers.

We are afraid that you may find yourself skimping on meals out of sheer exhaustion. That makes it especially important for you to have snacks that are easy to prepare, can be kept right on hand, and are full of nutrients but not too many calories. Low-fat yogurt is always good for a treat. Carrot sticks and celery sticks are easy to eat while you are breast-feeding and can be prepared ahead to have on hand. Apple slices on a plate, along with the cheese or perhaps spread with peanut butter, are delightful, if a bit more trouble to fix. A glass of V-8 juice can satisfy you while your baby nurses. If you want a quick treat that feels like junk food but is actually good for you, take out a bag of unbuttered microwave popcorn, and in just a few minutes you will have a hot treat to nibble on.

We suggest that you assign your partner the job of setting out a bowl of fruit, a full jug of water, and a glass each morning next to your favourite sport for nursing the baby. That way, every time you sit down to nurse during the day, you can reach out for a nutritious snack and a good drink of water and feel that someone is watching out for you even when you are home alone. Any fruit, especially apples and some varieties of pears, can be eaten with one hand and aren't even messy. Peaches and apricots are quite juicy to manage with one hand if you are holding the baby with the other, but they are so delicious and you can wipe up the juice with the towel you are using for burping the baby. Remember that raisins and other dried fruits are easy to keep on hand.

All that you eat goes not only into your body but also

influences your milk and therefore gets to your baby. If there are nutrients that you *don't* eat, your body will suffer the loss before the baby. It's therefore important to watch the quality of what you eat. It may seem a great number of calories, but you will need about 500 calories more than you normally require when you are nursing your baby. Vary your meals as much as you can, which is not an easy thing to do in the first weeks or even months after the birth of your baby. But as long as you get your calcium from cheese, milk, or yogurt one day, you could try to get your essential nutrients the next day from leafy green vegetables, or from fish, sardines, or canned tuna, if possible with the bones. Remember, what you eat will influence the consistency of your milk, and there may be certain foods that agree better with your baby than others.

The amazing fact is that your body will produce not only the right quantity of milk, but as your baby grows, it will also adjust the consistency to the changing needs of your child.

It is not too difficult to get the foods your body needs during this period. But here is a list of seven that are most likely to be deficient in a Western diet.

They are: iron, calcium, zinc, magnesium, vitamin D, vitamin E, and folic acid. All but iron are easy to take care of by choosing your foods with a bit more care than usual. You are probably getting enough vitamin D and calcium from drinking fortified low-fat milk. This is a good time in your life to eat plenty of bananas because they are a good source of potassium, which helps your body utilise the calcium you consume. Zinc is in meats, eggs, and whole grains.

Magnesium is in whole grains, beans, and nuts. Vitamin E is in wheat germ, nuts, many oils, and whole grains. Folic acid is in liver, spinach, nuts, and whole grains.

Notice how many of the deficits in the typical Western diet have occurred because we process the nutrients out of our grains. A switch to whole-grain breads and cereals goes a long way toward rectifying some of the problems of a typical Western diet.

While you are almost certainly taking an iron supplement, you may want to be aware of natural sources of the mineral also. Many of them are unpopular, like liver or spinach, or unfamiliar, like blackstrap molasses (which has as much iron in one tablespoon as you get from one and a half ounces of liver or half a cup of cooked spinach, not to mention its vitamin B_6 and its sweet taste). Perhaps the happiest way to make sure you are getting iron from your food is through a fresh salad of spinach leaves with peas, string beans, and cashew nuts. If you have a blender or food processor (and, perhaps, someone willing to wash it out for you), chopped chicken liver with cooked egg yolk crumbled on top would be a very special way to get your iron. Make up a big batch and you can have it available for a few days. Raisins, prunes, and dried apricots all have iron, as do sardines, shrimp, and tuna. Some cereals are enriched with iron. Check the labels.

Even though your baby is outside your uterus and active, you are still eating for two. You don't have to be as fearful that your life-style can adversely affect the child as you might have been during pregnancy, but as long as you are breast-feeding, everything that changes your body chemistry is likely to affect your milk and therefore have an influence on your baby.

The good nutrients get into your milk, but so do bad substances that you consume. We know that many women are convinced their baby gets irritable when they eat to much sugar and others who say their baby gets gas when they eat Brussels sprouts or broccoli. Ask any farmer; the quality and flavour of the milk produced by his cows is influenced by the grains they eat. Humans may be far more sophisticated and intellectual than cows, but the process of making milk is not that different. In each case, the mother creates a food that is designed for her own species.

Watch your baby at the breast. If he latches on, then pulls away and frets or fails to settle in to a meal, it may be because the taste of your milk does not suit him just now. What did you eat half an hour or so before that session of nursing? One unfortunate mum told us her newborn was fretful after a birthday party at which she enjoyed a large piece of chocolate cake; she is not the first to think that chocolate eaten by the mother can cause diarrhoea in the baby. Nervous and hyperactive babies may have received a dose of caffeine via their mothers' milk. We know a child who turned away from the breast while his mother was being treated with antibiotics for pneumonia. It was as though he just did not like the taste anymore.

We all know that during pregnancy great care is taken that the mother does not take any medication that may go through her bloodstream, through the placenta into the foetus. The taboos are numerous: no aspirin, no alcohol, no cigarettes, no antihistamines even as nose drops, no sleeping pills, no Valium. Should these restrictions be kept in place during breast-feeding, or are they only relevant during pregnancy? In general, they are real concerns. Many of the prohibitions of pregnancy should be extended through lactation.

Whenever you need any medication, you should balance benefit and risk. For many prescription drugs, even those that pass into the breast milk, benefit far outweighs the possibility of risk. Many popular antibiotics (for example, amoxicillin and ampicillin) pass into the breast milk in small quantities. It is theoretically possible that the baby might have an allergic reaction to the antibiotic, but the odds are slight and the benefit of treating a serious infection in the mother are great. Your health-care professionals will help you with these decisions.

In general, prescription drugs should be used with extra caution during breast-feeding. If they must be taken even though they pass into the breast milk, you should be in careful consultation with your physician about their possible effects on milk production or on your baby's well-being. In many cases, the drugs will pass through your system in a few hours. Both the amount of the drug and the length of time that it will appear in your milk vary widely from substance to substance. You can ask your doctor for details about any drug he prescribes, and you may be able to get further advice from your local group of La Leche League and the Association of Breast-feeding Mothers (see page 136).

Antihistamines are in a questionable area of risk. They seem to inhibit milk production and can make a baby drowsy. Aspirin does pass into breast milk, but the only impact on the baby is the theoretical but unproven possibility that it might affect blood clotting. Over-the-counter bronchodilators that contain ephedrine or epinephrine used by the mother can cause irritability in a breast-fed newborn. If you are troubled with asthma, be sure to check with your physician before taking any prescription or non-prescription medication. Many over-the-counter allergy-relief medicines and cough suppressants probably enter breast milk.

Birth-control pills contain oestrogen, which is naturally depressed during breast-feeding. A woman who takes oestrogen may find that her milk production is inhibited, but there does not seem to be any danger to the infant from the hormone passing through the breast milk. If you cannot switch to any other form of birth control, consider supplementing breast-feeding with formula or, in an older baby, solid foods if there is any evidence that he or she is not getting enough milk. If you must take the pill while breast-feeding, take one with the lowest possible dose of oestrogen and watch your baby's weight gain carefully.

We know that many young women take laxatives as a way to control their weight. This is a bad idea at any time, but especially now. If you find yourself constipated, there are more natural ways to get your bowels moving again. For example, you can eat more high-fibre cereals, prunes, figs, dried apricots, or, for some people, a hot liquid first thing in the morning. If none of those dietary modifications work, talk to your physician about the pros and cons of various laxatives. Some are safer than others.

Illegal substances are definitely a risk to a breast-fed baby not only because they appear in the breast milk, but also because they can affect the mother's competence to care for the baby. Alcohol is not as dangerous now as it was during pregnancy, when it passed directly from the mother's bloodstream to the baby's bloodstream and through his vulnerable brain and liver as they were just forming. During lactation, the alcohol passes from the mother's bloodstream to the milk. It then passes into the baby's stomach where it is digested, and therefore gets to the baby's brain and liver in less dangerous doses. Women have often been told to drink a glass of wine or beer while they breast-feed their baby; some say it stimulates the milk supply or facilitates the let-down reflex. However, that contented baby may actually be tipsy. A soft lullaby is a far healthier way to soothe him to sleep.

Alcohol passes through your system in hours. Marijuana and other drugs can linger for days. Many drug-treatment programmes tell lactating women not to breast-feed for three days after a lapse with cocaine because of the serious damage that can be done to a baby from that chemical in the milk.

Some people find it very difficult to eat sensibly or to stay away from unhealthy substances. If you have a history of eating disorders or weight fluctuation, you may be very nervous about your diet. If you have a history of substance abuse, you may be worried about hurting your baby. When in doubt, turn to others for help. Your community is sure to have weight-control counsellors and nutritionists as well as groups like AA (Alcoholics Anonymous) and NA (Narcotics Anonymous) (see page 136) to help you stay on track for a healthy life.

After the six-week checkup, you probably have your health provider's okay to exercise as much as you want. As at any time in your life, be sensible and build up your strength and endurance gradually. When you are breast-feeding, it is particularly important that you do not overexert yourself.

One study suggests that babies do not like the lactic acid produced in their mothers' bodies during vigorous exercises. They were fretful at the breast in nursing sessions after exercise class. This problem can be solved by expressing breast milk before class and saving it for later or for simply waiting sixty to ninety minutes or more before nursing the baby after class.

If you still have a good reserve of fat stored on your hips and thighs, you may be able to exercise without fear of nutritional depletion, but if you are already back to your pre-pregnancy weight while breast-feeding, remember that you need more calories and more nutrients than usual because you are feeding yourself and the baby. Be sensitive to your hunger and your thirst, for they are indications of your body's need.

There are also a few special considerations now. The most obvious is that your breasts are larger than usual and may be quite sensitive. We recommend that you wear a very good support bra so that you will be comfortable during vigorous activity. Many women find it uncomfortable to run or jump or perform any exercise that makes their breasts bounce, but others are quite comfortable. Walking and swimming are particularly good exercises at this time. Set your own pace and be sensitive to the unique responses of your body.

5
Weight Change Over the Childbearing Year

Most women have a healthy pregnancy and still have a store of potential energy for labour and breast-feeding while keeping their weight gain of pregnancy under 2½ stone (15.9 kg). Much of that weight will disappear gradually over the first nine months of the baby's life.

A women in excellent health who eats very nutritious foods can do well while gaining less weight than is generally recommended in guidelines for pregnancy, but she will have to work harder on her diet to get all the vitamins and minerals she and her baby need. A woman who is underweight when she conceives should gain more than the minimum recommendation; a women who is overweight when she conceives may be able to get away with putting on less.

If you tend to eat a diet of junk food, if you are a teenager and still growing yourself, if you carried twins or triplets, or if you went through several pregnancies spaced very closely together, you needed to be especially careful to get enough nutrients during pregnancy to keep up your strength after the birth. Similarly, if you exercised a great deal during the pregnancy, you needed more nutrients than the average woman. You should also know that if you smoked, drank alcohol, or used illicit substances that affected your metabolism, you and your baby were at greater risk of malnutrition and therefore would have special need of vitamins and minerals.

Busy professional women, single mothers, women on weight-loss diets, the underweight, and the overweight are targets of special medical concern during the childbearing year because if they are not eating a varied and nutritious diet, their health may suffer. If you fell into any of those categories during pregnancy, you may find that you are exhausted now, after the birth. Be especially careful to get the nutrition you need so that your recovery can be healthy and happy.

You may have decided to relax into the childbearing year rather than get involved in an elaborate nutritional analysis of all the food you ate during pregnancy. Or perhaps you thought, Oh, wow, now I'm going to get fat anyway, so I can eat everything I want! If so, you probably gained quite a bit of weight and will be interested in losing it over the next six months or so.

Here are the words of Maggie:

'I was craving all sorts of things during pregnancy, especially meat. I knew I didn't need French fries to help my baby grow, but I would let myself eat them and all sorts of other junk. Knowing it was wrong just made me more depressed, and so I'd eat more and feel even worse.'

Maggie finally joined a pregnancy support group and began a routine of daily relaxation to music. She did gain over 60 pounds during the pregnancy, but she and the baby were healthy and her eating patterns relaxed after the birth. You will hear from her later in this chapter as she describes the new relationship she developed to food while she was caring for her daughter.

We want to share with you the stories of three women whom we interviewed in depth. We have chosen these three because they are so distinctly different in their starting places and their outcomes. The first, Alice, was at her ideal weight before she became pregnant, but she gained 4 stone 9 pounds (29.5 kg) and had to work hard to lose it afterward. Six months after the birth, she weighed 15 pounds (6.8 kg) more than she had when she started. The second, Bonnie, was underweight when she decided to try to get pregnant. She had to gain weight to conceive and was plagued by fatigue after the birth, though she regained her original weight very quickly. The third, Carol, was about 15 pounds (6.8 kg) over her preferred weight when she discovered that she was going to have a baby. She gained 1 stone 12 pounds (11.8 kg) during the pregnancy and had lost 2 stone 3 pounds (14.1 kg) by the time her son was six months old. Here are their stories, in their own words.

ALICE

Alice is a tall, large-boned woman in her mid-thirties. At 5′10″, (1.78m), she weighed 10 stone 2 pounds (64.4 kg) and was a perfect size 12. For her, an ideal weight gain would have been 25–35 pounds (11.3–15.8 kg). When she decided to have a baby, she stopped smoking and drinking and started gaining weight before she even became pregnant.

'I immediately ate more because of giving up smoking. I became pregnant very quickly and was terribly nauseous for the first three months. The doctor told me to keep something in my stomach all the time, so I worked out a daily schedule consisting of breakfast at home of milk and raisin bran, then a second breakfast at work of a double egg/bacon/cheese sandwich, a large V-8 juice, and fruit salad; a snack of yogurt or a muffin at midmorning; a lunch of soup, sandwich and crisps; an early afternoon snack of fruit and a late afternoon snack of cereal or biscuits; and dinner of either chicken or steak, two vegetables, and mashed potatoes. He had given me the excuse I had been waiting for. I had kept my weight where it was by being careful. I had exercised a lot, swimming four times a week and walking the dog for an hour a day. Now I let go.

'In the first three months I was exhausted. I went swimming only once a week and walked the dog at a much slower pace. I gained 2 stone 10 pounds (17.2 kg). Obviously, I was doing a lot more than the doctor suggested. I was not just nibbling on things to keep something in my stomach. I was overeating.

'The nausea passed after three and a half months. Then I ate less and exercised more. I felt terrific. During months four to seven, I only put on half a stone (3.2 kg).

'In the last three months I put on weight again. I was still swimming two or three times a week up to two days before my son was born, but I had gained so much weight that I waddled when I walked. I weighed 14 stone 11 pounds (93.9 kg) and couldn't wait to have him.

'I spent two night in the hospital after Andy was born. I was exhausted and had no appetite, perhaps because of the Percocet they gave me. I didn't eat at all that first day, though they did bring in a dinner tray.

'I had it on my mind to lose weight right away and started watching what I ate immediately. Now I eat three meals and two light snacks a day. My meals are sensible: no mashed potatoes, sweets or butter; skim milk instead of whole milk; a half sandwich instead of a whole sandwich. My snacks are restricted to fresh fruit, raw vegetables, or non-fat yogurt. I have little time to make elaborate snacks anyway.

'I lost 2 stone 2 pounds (13.6 kg) in the first month. A lot of it was water. I have always retained a lot of water during my menstrual period, too.

'I am still breast-feeding and do not want to go on a crash diet. I lost ten pounds (4.5 kg) in the second month after giving birth. I am pretty active. I go to exercise class two times a week. It is not aerobic and doesn't burn calories, but it is a motivator and helps keep me on track and in touch with my body. I am eating lightly and carefully. I smoke a little now and drink half a glass of wine at night. I have found that I do not want to drink more than that because I am breastfeeding. Besides, I hate getting up in the night with the buzz of the alcohol wearing off.

'My husband does the cooking at night, which is a great help. The few times that I forgot to take a meal, it was horrible. I felt really shaky.

'Next time I get pregnant, I am going to work hard to keep my gain to 2 stone 2 pounds. I feel this extra weight is unnecessary work and trouble. I am eager to be able to slip back into my regular clothes instead of having to wear my husband's shirts and stretch pants.'

One month after giving birth, Alice's weight was 12 stone 9 pounds (80.3 kg). Alice continued to lose weight. When we last spoke to her, her baby was six months old and Alice weighed 11 stone 3 pounds (71.2 kg). She said she was 'not dieting but eating sensibly'. She thought it would take her another two months to get to her pre-pregnancy weight.

BONNIE

Bonnie has always been very slender. At 5′6″ (1.68m), she weighed only 8 stone 5 pounds (53.1 kg). She had trouble conceiving the first few months that she tried, and the doctor suggested that she gain a little extra weight. She weighed 8 stone 8 pounds (54.4 kg) when she conceived. A weight gain of 28–40 pounds (12.7–18.1 kg) would be recommended for Bonnie. Since she was so close to normal, she could try for the lower end of that range.

Here are her words:

'At the very beginning of my pregnancy, I had a spurt of weight gain. It evened out at five or six months without my changing anything at all. I ate normally but added cheese to my diet. Throughout the pregnancy, I seemed to have spurts. Sometimes my appetite would become huge and I'd eat as much as I wanted. My husband encouraged me, saying that I shouldn't worry about it because the baby needed it. Then I would have a period where I wasn't particularly hungry and I would eat less. I got up to just over 10 stone (64 kg), which was a gain of twenty-four pounds over what I consider my normal weight.

'Labour lasted seven hours. I had an epidural and had to push for two hours, but the doctors and nurses were all very responsive and took good care of me. Bobbie weighed seven pounds eight ounces (3.4 kg) and nursed in the delivery room. I was pleased that he seemed to know just what to do. Then he was taken to the nursery and we went to our room. My husband slept at the hospital.

'That first day, I felt like I was still pregnant, but

when I put my hand down on my abdomen, it felt flatter. I ate when they brought me food because I was afraid I was losing weight and I wanted to be able to produce milk. When Bobbie suckled, I could feel my uterus getting smaller through the contractions.

'I didn't do any exercises in the hospital, though I did deep breathing to relax in bed. I have always done meditation and kept that up.

'Two days later, the doctor said Bobbie had a high bilirubin, indicating that he had jaundice. I went home, but he had to stay in the hospital another three days to receive light treatments. While he was there, they fed him with formula to get him to pass stools. Whether it is because of that or something else, I don't know, but I have had trouble with breast-feeding. I have had to use a system of supplementation to get him to gain weight at a normal rate.

'When I first got home from the hospital I weighed 9 stone 4 pounds (59 kg). Then I just saw the pounds melt away, down to 9 stone (57.2 kg) then 8½ stone (54 kg). Seven weeks after giving birth I was back to where I was before I even tried to get pregnant, back to 8 stone 5 pounds.

'My sister came to stay with me after the baby was born. She is a big La Leche League advocate and kept saying, "You've got to eat, eat, eat." I have never had a big appetite and have always been a slow eater, but I am also aware of the importance of good food and would like to have time to eat more.

'I am still trying to get used to my baby's rhythms. I give him the 3 a.m. feeding in the rocking chair, but at six I am so tired I bring him to bed and we both fall asleep again there.

'The baby was not gaining well at first. I moved him gradually from the supplemental system to complete breast milk. I feel you have to give a lot in life and that I am going to have to produce a lot to satisfy him. I make sure each day to have a good breakfast of nutritious food; yogurt and fruit or cereal or eggs and toast. My husband usually cooks supper and I almost always get fish or chicken. I snack on fruit and cheese throughout the day.'

Bonnie's weight was low at the beginning of the pregnancy and continues to be low after the pregnancy. Weight loss is not a problem for her. To the contrary, her sister's words 'Eat, eat, eat' ring through her mind as she dedicates herself to keeping up her energy and breast-feeding her baby.

CAROL

Carol had her second boy when she was forty. Her first son had been born twelve years earlier. Before that pregnancy, she weighed 10 stone (63.5 kg), a normal weight for a woman 5′8″ (1.7m) tall. She gained 2½ stone (15.9 kg) in that pregnancy, lost 10 pounds (4.5 kg) in the early days after the birth but did not try to lose any more. Here are her words:

'At first I was surprised at my figure. I felt like it wasn't me. I hadn't got into being a mother.

'When he went on solid foods at six months, I dieted a little and lost another ten pounds (4.5 kg), but I never made an effort to lose the rest. I was breast-feeding, so I thought the weight would just come off.

'I was not happy about the extra weight, but I didn't want to have to focus on food and eating. My older sister is obsessed with food and plans everything she eats. I don't want my life to be ruled like that. I'm always in the mood to eat if I see a piece of cake. I don't like to diet, because I feel deprived. I'll bypass something I really want one day and then I'll take two of them the next day.

'Three years ago, I got a new job that was more sedentary than anything I'd done before. Working there, I put on weight again until I was up to 11 stone 6 pounds. (72.5 kg). That put me about 1½ stone (9 kg) over the weight I had been before my first pregnancy. I had thought about the possibility of having another baby and had vaguely thought that I should lose ten pounds (4.5 kg) before getting pregnant, but when I actually decided I wanted to go ahead, the weight became irrelevant. I got pregnant within a month of deciding.

'My feeling is that when you're pregnant, it is not a time to do strange things to your body. I took prenatal vitamins and I didn't exercise much. I feel that pregnancy is a time to slow down. I didn't gain enough in the first three months, but by the fifth month I had gained ten pounds (4.5 kg). I gained 1 stone 12 pounds (11.8 kg) in all. In my first pregnancy, it was packets of biscuits when I wanted them; this time I was more mature. I always ate three well-balanced meals a day plus dessert.

'Now Charles is ten weeks old. I lost 1 stone 2 pounds (7.3 kg) in the first month doing nothing. I don't know how much more I've lost since. I know how to diet, but right now I don't want to do anything to hurt Charles and he's still breast-feeding.

'I have been eating desserts, and loving every minute of it, but now I'm planning to cut out sweets. I've joined a Mother and Baby class, which is a session of exercises with the baby, and I'm about to start going to a gym. I know I'll enjoy that once I get into it. Now that he is sleeping through the night, I have enough energy to take on things like that. The first two months I couldn't possibly have done it. I had to conserve my energy and not do any more than the minimum.

'Everything has been easier this time around. With the second child, you know there will be an end to it. My husband has been very helpful, shopping and doing things around the house. I thought of hiring someone for the first few weeks, but I couldn't find anybody. Now I have a baby-sitter who comes two afternoons a week, so I can pay attention to my own needs as well as the baby's.'

Two weeks after she started exercising, Carol learned that

she had a minor condition that required surgery. She did not have to stay in the hospital very long, but she did have to restrict her activities for the next six weeks. Fortunately, her relaxed attitude helped her adjust to the disruption in her weight-loss regime. 'I figure it took me nine months to put on the weight, why shouldn't it take nine months to take it off?' she said to us when her baby was six months old. At that time, her weight was 11 stone 11 pounds (74.8 kg) and she had just resumed her visits to the gym. Charles was taking solid foods as well as breast-feeding. 'I'm not in any rush,' she said, 'My friend Maria has a fifteen-month-old, and she has just reached the point of needing a whole new wardrobe, a size smaller than she wore before she got pregnant. She's my role model! I figure Mother Nature know what she's doing. There has got to be a reason why we put on that weight. Right now, I just want to keep my strength up.'

We are all tempted to compare ourselves to your friends and neighbours. Try to remember that you are unique. Your body has its own metabolism and its own pace of doing things. You will hear stories of women who magically lost all the weight gained from pregnancy within the first six weeks, and you will hear just as many stories—or maybe even more—about women who never lost their pregnancy gain. Which will you be? That depends on your particular body and on your patterns of eating and exercising. Again we want to reiterate the importance of establishing a pattern for life. Before you had a baby, you might have eaten sensibly

Weight Change Over the Childbearing Year

and exercised regularly. Now you don't have as much time to pay attention to these details of your life. You must establish new patterns that take into consideration the new demands.

You may be a woman who has had a pattern of extreme weight fluctuations. You may have had periods of radical dieting and periods of bingeing. You, too, must struggle to find a new way. The old pattern was not good for you. Each time you went on a radical regime to lose fat, you lost muscle mass as well. Your metabolism altered to get used to your low calorie count. Then you started to eat again and your body converted the new calories to fat. It's a proven fact that the cycle of losing and gaining the same ten pounds (4.5 kg) is unhealthy.

Whatever your life-style was, it is bound to be different now. Adjustments are necessary for your new life with the baby. Sometimes, motherhood can change your life in unexpected ways.

Listen to Maggie's experience watching her daughter eat:

'At first it amazed me to see that she stopped eating when she was satisfied. I saw her pure greed, how simply she enjoyed eating. She sucked so vigorously, the milk dripping down her chin, and then when she was done, she simply stopped. I loved her sense of shameless hunger combined with her sensible stopping when she had enough. I wish I would find a way to help her keep her healthy relationship to food.

'Right now I am trying to lose weight, and the doctor

has put me on a diet in which I am not allowed to eat any sugar. In the past, if somebody had said 'You can never eat sweets again,' I would have been desperate. Now that I have learned about eating from my daughter, I know that it isn't the sweets that matter. If I crave something, I think, What do you really want? It's never really candy. Sometimes I want love; sometimes I'm angry and afraid to express it; sometimes I'm frustrated over the details of my life or in a conflict with my mother. When I figure out what it is and what I'm feeling, I find I can let the sweets go.

'I trust my body to tell me when I need food and when I have had enough. I wasn't like that before I had a baby.'

Becoming a mother can be a transformational experience, but you are still the same person underneath. Take it gradually, one step at a time. If you expect too much of yourself, you will go to extremes and lose a quick 5 pounds (2.3 kg) then gain them right back again. Work toward a lifestyle solution, not a recurring problem.

We feel that you should be as realistic as possible about preparing meals that feel 'normal' to you. A radical departure from your old style might keep you interested for a short time, but you need to have eating patterns to last you throughout your life. If you want to lose weight after you have a baby, you will also find yourself concerned about the gradual weight that you tend to gain with age. Use this year as a time of your life to gradually shape your eating patterns for the long haul. Try to get away from the idea that you have to shed a pound or half a kilo a week. Accept the fact that you are involved in a long, gradual process. Stay with it; do not give up. Don't look for the instant gratification of weight falling off as it did in the first six weeks after giving birth. Retrain yourself to a life-style that includes healthy eating, good exercise, time for your own recreation, and responsible care of your children, not to mention the probability of your own employment outside the home. This is a tall order! But let's look at some simple shifts that you can make in your eating habits at home, shifts that you can share with your whole family (except the baby, who will have to wait a bit).

As we said in chapter 3, if you are interested in losing weight, you must eliminate junk foods that are overladen with fat and sweet treats that are loaded with sugar. What will you substitute for these treats that will be as satisfying to your tastes and just as easy to get when you are tired and hungry?

If you have always cooked hamburgers at least one evening a week, you can simply switch to ground turkey and change from a traditional bun of empty calories to a whole-grain bun that provides nutrition as well as taste. If you adore ketchup, we won't suggest that you eliminate it entirely from your burger, but try to cut your amount in half. Substitute boiled potatoes with low-fat margarine for the chips or, even better, prepared baked potatoes. You can bake several at a time, then reheat them one by one in the microwave and top them with non-fat yogurt instead of butter or soured cream.

Whenever possible, eat foods that are almost identical to your favourites. Have a milk shake, but use skimmed milk. Have a soda, but make sure it is a diet soda or simply soda water flavoured with a little fruit juice. Have an omelette, but use only the white of the eggs and as little oil as possible.

In your attempts to serve low-calorie versions of your usual meals, don't make the mistake of eating things that are empty of both calories and nutrition. Dietary foods on the supermarket shelves often fall into this category. Remember, you still need all those important nutrients for health, particularly as you are caring for a baby. While a diet soda is okay, a glass of skimmed milk is better. Both give you fluids, but only the milk gives you calcium and protein. Similarly, a dietetic coffee cake may seem like a comfort food, but a whole-grain muffin has more to offer your body and is worth the calories.

This is a great time to take charge of your eating habits. Now that you are a mother, you may feel that you are doing what is best for your child and find that it is much easier than you expected to give up alcohol and–if you smoked–tobacco, and to cut fat and sugar from your diet. You may be proud and happy to switch from greasy crisps to unsalted popcorn, for that is a badge of what a good mother you are. You may go from whole milk to skimmed, from cheese to tofu, from pork chops to grilled fish. If you liked the ease of opening a can of spaghetti hoops for lunch, you will find that it is just as easy and far more delicious to open a can of salmon with bones packed in water (a fabulous source of calcium) to eat with whole-grain bread or a baked potato.

On the other hand, some of you may be surprised to discover that you are having a harder time controlling yourself than you could have imagined. You may know that you are supposed to be sensible and to eat well, but you are too busy or too tired to manage it. You may feel that you have worked so hard that you deserve some indulgence. You've given up your job, you are alone at home for long stretches devoting yourself to someone who can't even thank you for it. Many of us turn to food when we are feeling sorry for ourselves. We overeat for comfort, especially when we feel deprived or guilty or overburdened. For some mysterious reason, the most comforting foods are those that, like a rejecting mother, seem to promise more than they can deliver. Danish pastries, crisps, ice cream, chips–they fill you up, then let you down.

The feelings of resentment, exhaustion, and frustration that come up in the early months of taking care of a baby are often a great shock to a new mother. You want to be patient and loving and in control of your emotions and of your life, but somehow the postnatal period (which stretches on for months, or even years) is harder than you expected. All your good intentions seem to dissolve before the temptation of a container of ice cream or a bag of crisps. When the baby's fussing gets on your nerves and you begin to wonder how you are going to keep your temper, get yourself away from the biscuit tin. Pack up the baby. Go for a walk or for a ride in the car. Either one will probably put the baby to sleep. Get out of the house, or invite a friend in. Don't let anger or frustration get the upper hand.

There are so many good excuses for not being able to eat well. Louise told us why she seemed to have so much trouble losing weight after she had her second child:

'Some days I don't have time to get lunch for myself, or I snack on junk. And losing weight is not just a matter of limiting food. I have to exercise, too, and the health clubs in the city do not have babysitters, so I can't go.

'If I had full-time live-in help, then I would join a health club and probably be able to get back in shape as quickly as the first time, but I have part-time help, and it is hard to feel comfortable leaving two kids with a sitter who is there only part-time.

'I feel as if I'm stuck in a body that is not toned. To you I may look in shape, but I can't find time to exercise at home. Beyond even getting in shape, I just want to get so that I can sometimes feel rested during the day.'

It's not one thing that keeps Louise from eating as well as she would like or exercising as much as she feels she should. She is overwhelmed with her life right now. She will have to get her schedule under control before she can undertake the secondary task of losing weight.

We have known women who solved the dilemma of finding free time for themselves by forming a child-care cooperative or joining a mothers' network or finding a relative who will look after the children two mornings a week.

Those of you who are lucky enough to live in the suburbs may find that you do have a local health club that provides child care. Some even have exercise classes for older children, which run concomitantly with the Mother and Baby classes that incorporate the infant into the exercise regime of the mother. And of course you can exercise at home with your baby, turning it into a game, toning your body, and entertaining your children at the same time.

Exercise alone will not solve the problem of losing weight. You also need a balanced personal life that includes a sensible pattern of eating. It would be helpful to work out a programme for breakfast, lunch, and dinner that would provide a balanced diet without putting too much strain on your time. You should not be bothered with fancy cooking or an elaborate nutritional analysis unless cooking is your favourite hobby and relaxation.

Getting out of the house and meeting other adults may be just as important to your ability to get back to feeling like yourself and returning to your pre-pregnancy figure as any other factor. Find some way to get child care so that you can be free to enjoy yourself. Studies show that women who return to work lose weight faster than those who stay at home with their children. Is this because they get more exercise at work? We think it is just as likely that their contact with the outside world changes their feelings about themselves and changes their eating habits.

6

Putting It All Together

We live in a society that puts forward an ideal of thin women, an ideal that does not include the changing shape of motherhood. Purely physiologically speaking, it is essential that a woman who is to feel good about herself throughout her childbearing years be able to accept an image of the fertile, rounded woman.

Judith told us about her experience of visiting a friend who had just had a baby:

'When I picked up Sally's baby, I was anticipating that sensation I had had fifteen years before, with my own child, that wonderful fit of the newborn against my chest, but when I drew him up to me, I was amazed to discover that it didn't feel right. At first, I thought that it was because he was too thin and frail, but then I understood that it was because *I* was too thin. *I* was the one who had lost the body of a new mother, the body designed to connect so intimately with a newborn baby.'

Judith has none of that soft maternal padding left. She is very slender now, a trait that she says she shares with all the members of her family.

Accepting a more rounded, motherly image of yourself is not at all the same as letting yourself go or becoming fat and sloppy. We are talking about the slight padding that goes along with pregnancy and lactation. Even if you don't breast-feed, you may retain some of the softness and roundness you have acquired during childbearing, although if your body type is slender, you may lose that roundness over the years.

If you hadn't been eating carefully before, you should learn to do so now. Your health is not just your own concern, but your child's as well. We all know that we don't function well if we don't get enough sleep and if we are hungry.

We cannot overemphasise the importance of learning to pay attention to your own body. Your body needs different amounts of food at different times in your life. Right now, after giving birth, you need more calories, more nutrients, and more fluids than usual.

Because of the stress of parenthood, we suggest that you try to have something to eat at regular times during the day. If you wait until your body reminds you to eat, you may have become depleted. In the postnatal period, it is helpful to make sure that you have at least a small amount of food regularly during the day so that you always have a bit of energy in reserve. Pick up on the early signs of hunger and pick up on the early signs of being full. Both you and your baby need to learn to regulate your eating. After all, one of the important tasks for the baby in the first year of life is to learn to eat and sleep in rhythms that suit the entire family.

If you think you should eat a certain amount no matter

Putting It All Together

what else is going on, you will gain weight as you age. If you eat in response to actual hunger and are sensitive to the needs of your body, it will be easier for you to eat less when your body needs less. For example, Judy was told that her baby was not growing enough during her second trimester of pregnancy. Her doctor told her to drink a special high-calcium, high-protein milk shake with breakfast each morning. She needed those extra calories for the baby's growth at the end of pregnancy but didn't need them any more after giving birth.

'When I got home from the hospital, I was craving those milk shakes that I'd been drinking during the pregnancy, but I didn't let myself have them.'

Judy went on to talk about her feelings as the mother of a four-month-old baby.

'I feel so insecure. I feel judged if anybody says they do it differently. I think all new mothers need a lot or reassurance, to be told we are doing things right. I also think we should baby ourselves. Maybe in the past I would have done that by eating junk food or by making a pig of myself. Now I try to do it in a way that I won't have to pay for later. Like getting a baby-sitter and getting out on my own, or asking my husband to give me a massage, or by taking a long bath while the baby sleeps.'

Judy is quite right. The insecurity of new mothers is an

almost universal part of their experience. Now that so many of us raise our children far from our family of origin, we may not have sources of support and advice. In fact, child abuse and neglect are associated with social isolation. You need love and attention from others. While you are nurturing the child, you must be sure to find people around you who will be nurturing the new mother–you!

Molly told a typical story of an insecure new mum. She was pushing her six-month old in the pram through Hyde Park in London. An older woman came up to her and said, 'Oh, my dear, you have that baby so bundled up! Let it breathe.' Molly promptly removed the baby's woollen cap and continued on her way. Ten minutes later, she was waiting for a pedestrian light to change when a woman standing next to her said, 'Really, how could you have that child out without a hat!'

What is a new mother to do? You cannot possibly follow all of the contradictory advice.

One of the common surprises of parents is the way in which they find themselves thinking of their own mothers. Some of you may have vowed in adolescence that you would never do the terrible things that your mother did to you. Now that you are a mother yourself, you may develop more compassion for the stress that your mother was experiencing. You may find yourself doing exactly those things you swore you would never do. This can be terribly depressing. If you were often angry at your mother, you may worry that your own child will not love you. Turn to your baby at such a moment and realise that he or she will indeed love you.

Putting It All Together

Maggie describes her experience:

> 'Mothering has taught me the transformational power of babies. There are times when I'll start to worry. Will Lucy love me as much as she loves the baby-sitter? When I feel that, I say to myself, 'Just get down on the floor and play with her. Then she will love you because she has fun with you.' When I do that, I know that I am not like my own mother. She never played with us kids. I grew up being sedentary and solitary. When I was a teenager, my mother said, 'You would look so much better if you lost ten pounds (4.5 kg). Why don't you go on a diet?' If Lucy were to have a weight problem, I'd say, 'Let's go and play tennis!' Now she is only six months old, but I try to play physically with her. I want her to be active in her body, so each time that she is awake and alert, I try to engage her in some physical play.'

Maggie is not saying she does not love her mother. In fact, she is very close to her, especially now that she has a baby. What Maggie is doing is trying to break the cycle of a particular style of parenting. She knows that she learned an unhealthy relationship to food in her childhood, and she is creating a healthy pattern now, both for herself and for her daughter.

This realisation of what happened to you in childhood frees you to create your own pattern with yourself and your child. It is a way of liberating yourself from certain ideas you have carried with you since early childhood. You may fear that your new choices will alienate you from your parents. It is more likely that they will be proud and delighted to see you growing as a happy and creative adult. They do not want you to be locked into mistakes they may have made.

Over the early months and years with your child, you will have to evolve your own personal style of parenting, but this will not happen unaided. Your partner, your friends, your paediatrician, and your family members will all have opinions. Sometimes you may feel they are not very helpful, but remember, you have the right to reject their advice if it doesn't suit you. They can tell you what they think, but in the end you must trust your own feelings. As you gain more experience, it will grow easier to have this trust in yourself.

A mothers' support group can help you have a place where you can talk about your feelings and compare your mothering style with that of other women. You can discuss the pros and cons in a place that is free from judgment. Especially if you do not have friends or relatives with children close in age to yours, it is important to seek out a place where you can talk. If you do not have a natural social group for such conversations, call M.A.M.A. (Meet a Mum Association) or CRYSIS (see page 136). People won't come to your house to find you. You must go out to reach them. Go to the park with your baby in the pram. Go to a Mother and Baby class. Attend classes on parenting. You have to find your own solutions for the concerns of parenting, but it is best to do this in conversation with others. The activities will help you feel better about yourself and will keep you from a sedentary life at home, close to your refrigerator.

Putting It All Together

This trust in your own style of parenting is related to an ability to be able to feel secure and to know what is going on inside—not only inside your mind and your feelings, but also inside your body. Overeating may be a habit that is unrelated to physical need. If you are able to eat when hungry and stop when full, you will find you are regulating your own diet appropriately for your own needs. This is easier to say than to actually do. When you are overwhelmed with new responsibilities and unfamiliar tasks, anxious, or exhausted, you may forget to pay attention to your body.

Deep relaxation exercises help counteract the stress of the postnatal period. Some of you may turn to traditional meditation techniques, as Bonnie did from day one, although frankly we would be amazed to hear of many new mothers who actually had the time to do this. The disruption of your schedule can lead to poor eating and to constipation. We use the expression 'Staying regular' to refer to bowel function. Interestingly, the time after giving birth is a time when it is particularly difficult to stay regular in any way, even eating or sleeping. Try to have enough help with child care so that your fundamental bodily needs can be taken care of. Maybe you will get only ten minutes when your partner is at home to deal with your private needs alone, but do take at least that.

Some women find it helpful to lie quietly for a short period, listening to relaxing music. We both find that a session of stretching and breathing exercises helps us become aware of our bodies and become revitalised.

Our main message in this book about how to lose weight after having a baby is that you must be patient. We know

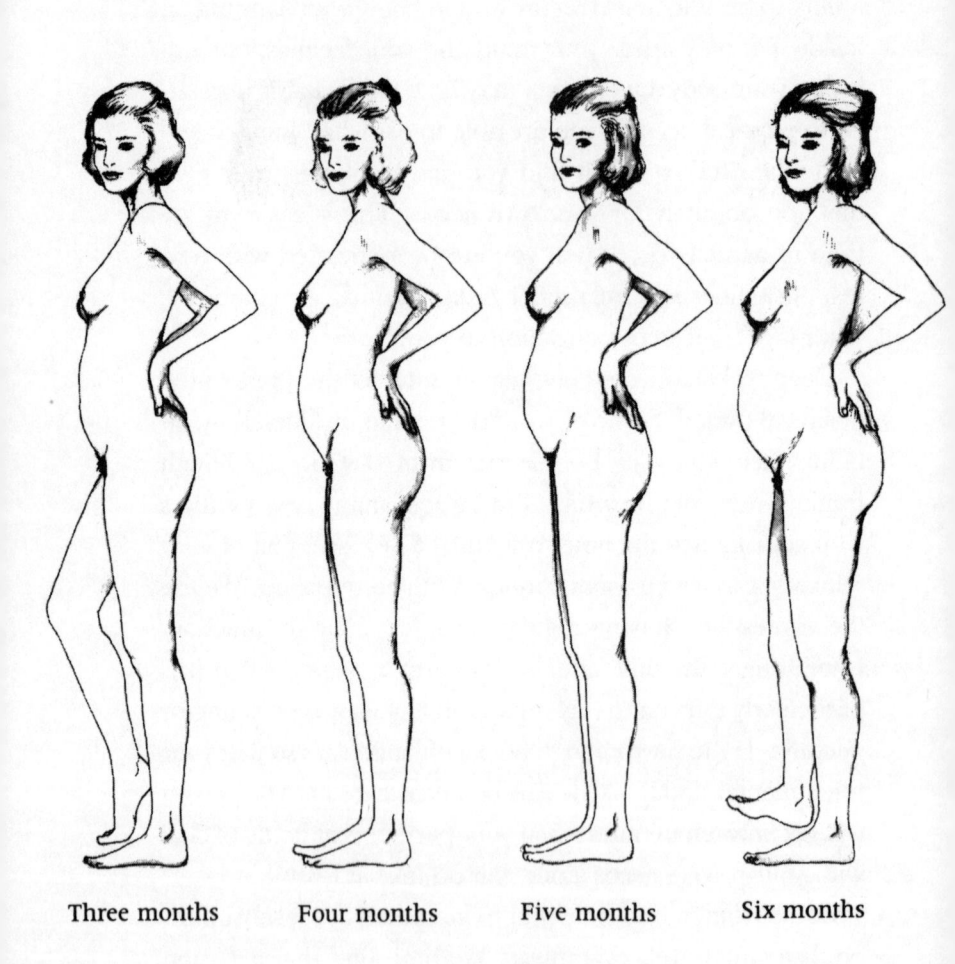

Three months   Four months   Five months   Six months

WEIGHT GAIN DURING PREGNANCY

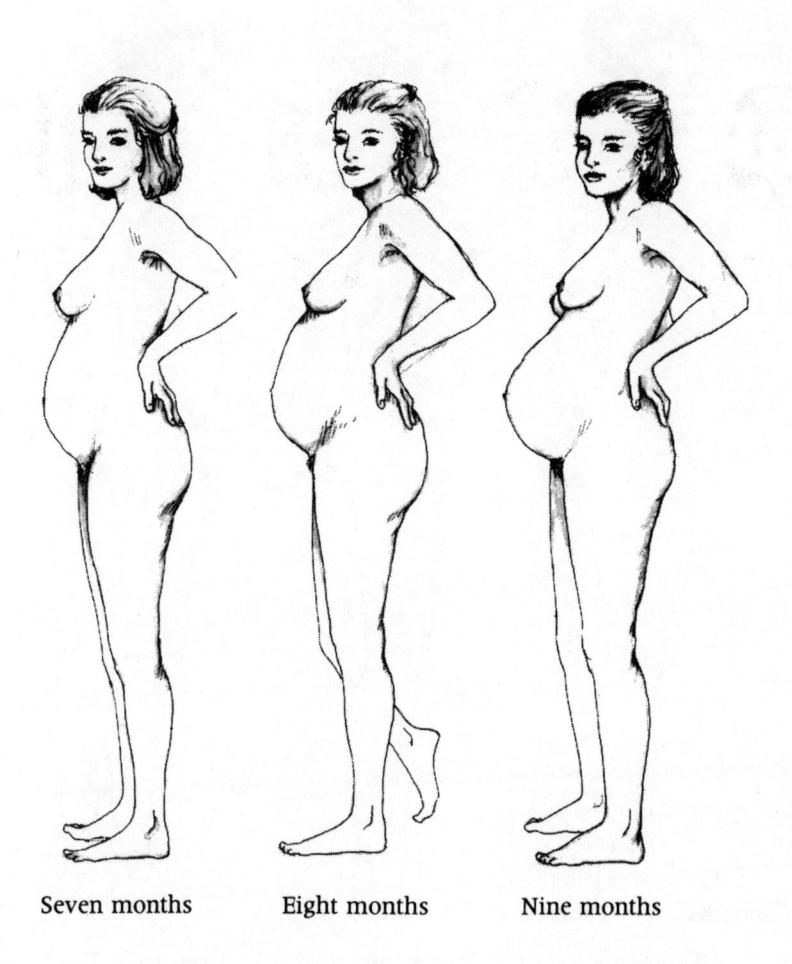

Putting It All Together

Seven months   Eight months   Nine months

WEIGHT GAIN DURING PREGNANCY

Losing Weight After Pregnancy

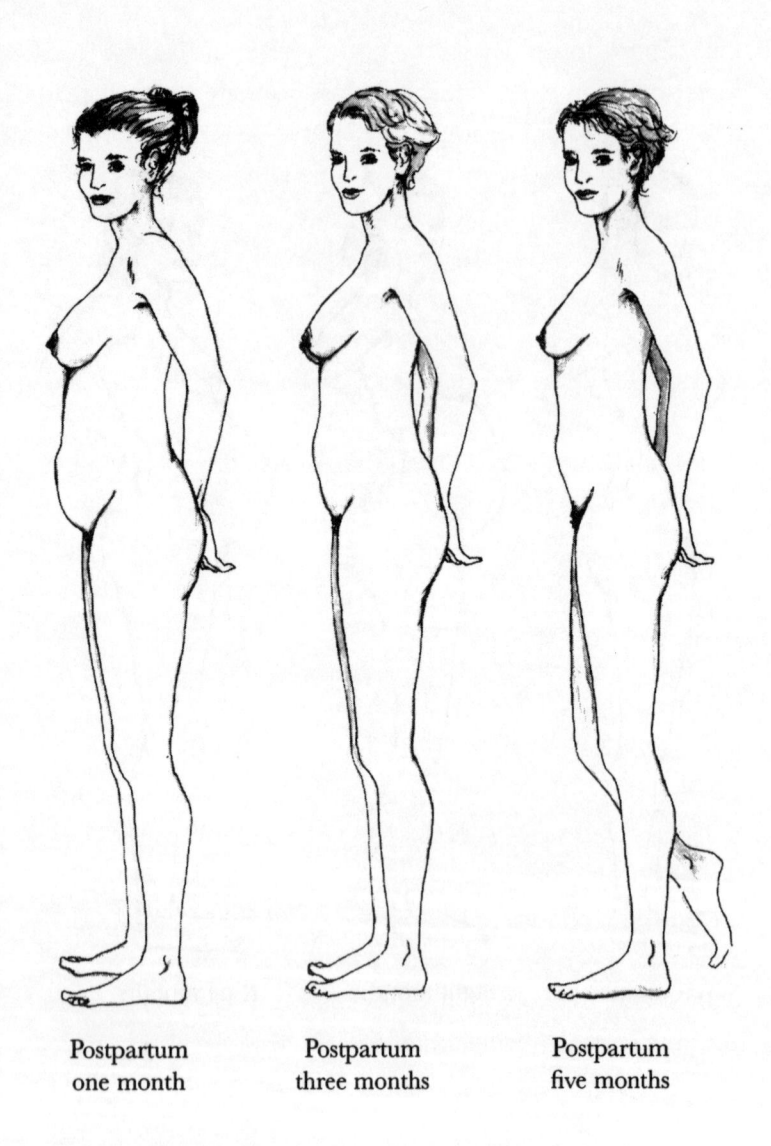

Postpartum one month   Postpartum three months   Postpartum five months

WEIGHT LOSS AFTER PREGNANCY

that is hard to do. By telling you to relax and accept your maternal body, we are going against fashion, and fashion is a very powerful influence. If you want to be elegant, you will have to rely on your own sense of colour and style, not on your mannequin-like figure.

These years with babies and toddlers in the house make special demands on your wardrobe as well as on your body. No matter how sweet the baby, it will need to burp. No matter how adorable the toddler, it will delight in mud and mess.

Both of us have lived through the gradual transition from being absorbed in the role of 'mum' to regaining that sense of being 'me'. Elisabeth's moment of independence came when she realised she could go to the supermarket with Peter not in a sling or a pram but walking on his own like a companion with whom she could discuss the errands of the day. Libby remembers her excitement when her youngest child started school and she went to buy the first silk blouse she had dared to wear in years.

Don't despair. Someday your babies will be big and your body will be your own. You can diet and exercise as you please. But we hope that you will continue to eat sensibly. When you can no longer say that you are doing it for the baby's sake, we hope that you will have learned to do it for your own sake; your health and well-being are as important as anybody's.

HELPFUL ORGANISATIONS

Association of Breast-feeding Mothers
26 Holmshaw Close
London SE26 5PN
Tel: 0181-788 4769

Association for Post-Natal Illness
25 Jerdan Place
London SW6 1BE
Tel: 0171-386 0868

British Diabetic Association
10 Queen Ann Street
London W1M 0BD
Tel: 0171-323 1531

Caesarian Support Group
c/o 7 Green Street
Willingham
Cambridgeshire CB4 5JA
Tel: 01954 60630

CRYSIS
B.M. Crysis
London WC1N 3XX
Tel: 0171-404 5011
(Support for parents of babies who cry excessively)

Gingerbread
35 Wellington Street
London WC2E 7BN
Tel: 0171-240 0953
(Help and advice for single parents)

La Leche League of Great Britain
BM 3424
London WC1N 3XX
Tel: 0171-242 1278
(Information and help on breastfeeding)

MAMA (Meet-a-Mum Association)
17 Hilton Village
Hilton
Inverness
Tel: 01463 234224

Narcotics Anonymous
UK Service Office, Tel: 0171-272 9040
(Check phone book for local branch details)

The National Childbirth Trust
Alexandra House
Oldham Terrace
Acton
London W3 6NH
Tel: 0181–992 8637
(branches all over the country)

National Council for One Parent Families
225 Kentish Town Road
London NW5 2LX
Tel: 0171–267 1361

Parentline
Rayfa House
57 Hart Road
Thundersley
Essex SS7 3PD
Tel: 01268 757077
(Organisation for parents under stress)

Parents Anonymous (London)
6 Manor Gardens
London N7 6LA
Tel: 0171–263 8918

Working Mothers Association
77 Holloway Road
London N7 8J7
Tel: 0171–700 5771